W H E N

I T ' S

C A N C E R

WHEN

IT'S

CANCER

THE 10 ESSENTIAL

STEPS TO FOLLOW

AFTER YOUR DIAGNOSIS

Toni Bernay, PhD, and Saar Porrath, MD
Founders of the Porrath Foundation for Cancer Patient Advocacy

Printed in the United States of America
Rodale Inc. makes every effort to use acid-free ∞, recycled paper ♻.

Interior design by Drew Frantzen
Cover design by Gavin Robinson

Library of Congress Cataloging-in-Publication Data

Bernay, Toni.
   When it's cancer : the 10 essential steps to follow after your diagnosis / Toni Bernay and Saar Porrath.
      p.   cm.
   Includes index.
   ISBN-13 978–1–57954–823–0 paperback
   ISBN-10 1–57954–823–7 paperback
   1. Cancer—Popular works. I. Porrath, Saar. II. Title.
RC263.B45 2006
616.99'4075—dc22   2005031250

Distributed to the trade by Holtzbrinck Publishers

2 4 6 8 10 9 7 5 3 1 paperback

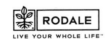

We inspire and enable people to improve their lives and the world around them

For more of our products visit **rodalestore.com** or call 800-848-4735

To our children

Mitch, Ellen, and Matt

Laura and Randy

and our grandchildren

Evan, Tessa, and Mia

with our love and appreciation for hanging in through the dark days,

celebrating the victories, and adding the laughter of children to our lives

CONTENTS

ACKNOWLEDGMENTS

This book has been a long journey—a journey that began with Saar's illness. Through it, he discovered his desire to share his knowledge and expertise as a radiologist and radiation and breast oncologist, as well as his ideas on patient-physician partnerships, with the public. Over time, his focus sharpened on his Personal Cancer Management System (PCMS) and his skills as a cancer patient advocate. His mission was to provide vital information to those who need it most: cancer patients and their loved ones.

As Saar's journey progressed, I joined him, providing the personal advocate's perspective along with additional cancer management tools, psychological insights, and case studies from cancer patients in my own practice who benefited from the PCMS. So many others made essential contributions as well; without their collective energy and wisdom, this book would not exist.

Saar wanted to be sure to thank our family and friends who encouraged and supported us as we wrote. I thank these same wonderful people, who helped me to stay the course through my mourning and through my own illness: Mitch Bernay, Ellen and Matt Lord, Laura and Randy Chalfin, Hedria Lunken, JoAnne and Lee Weisel, Ellen and Irwin Frankel, Gabe Hortobagyi, Sheldon and Karen Goodkind, Connie and Len Davis, Elliot Kajan, Ross Arbiter, and Margot Winchester.

Thanks to Jack Miles, whose literary talents, friendship, and spirituality so informed our writing; to Jeremy Tarcher for his sage advice; to the members of the Porrath Board who cheered me and brainstormed ideas with me: Elliot (again), Don Stolar, Faye Miller, Sandy Haber, Mimi West, and David Wellisch (who also served as cancer patient advocate for Saar and me); and to the wonderful women (and their spouses) who fed me, put up with my complaints, made suggestions, and kept pushing: Sondra Goldstein, Berta Davis, Elaine Rodino, Helen Grusd, Jana Martin, Helene Feldman, Lilli Friedland, Sabrina Mansfield, Dorothy Cantor, Laura Barbanel, Harriet Bay, Gayle Rodgers, and Bronya Galef.

To Saar's and my medical family from Cedars-Sinai Medical Center, UCLA, USC/Norris Comprehensive Cancer Center, M.D. Anderson Cancer Center, and St. John's Regional Medical Center, who added much information to the book: Paul O'Dea, Dan Stepan, Greg Sarna, Brian Durie, Ray Alexanian, Gabe Hortobagyi, Ron Thompson, Leon Bender, Mitch Komaiko, Ron Grusd, Dale Rice, Ed Wolin, Peter Rosen, Carey Strom, and Joe Sugarman.

Thanks to Lydia Mouzaka and the European contingent of the American Society of Breast Disease and the International Society of Senology (Breast); to Keith Hoshal, Eileen Brown, Fe San Angel, Harumi Mankarios, and Arpy Nahabedia, oncology nurses extraordinaire; and to Alan Schwab, part of the Mayberry on Bedford Drive community, who always went the extra mile when medications were needed.

To our complementary medicine friends, who helped energize us body, mind, and soul for the duration of this project: Jeff Rochford, David Wong, Michael Waterhouse, David Allen, and Lobsang Rapgay; to Maria DeBoer for her wonderful hands; and to Amberly Brown for her cheerleading and strength building.

Thanks to my "science" readers, Ken Schueler and Ron Thompson, who kept me honest.

To my agent, Carol Mann, who had faith in the book despite it being a little close to home; to my editor, Susan Berg, who struggled with me to marry personal and professional material; to Arthur Morey, who gave me so many good words and so much support; and to Mary Sutherland, my wonderful assistant, who sweated out this process with grace and charm, sharing her insights as we burned the midnight oil together.

INTRODUCTION

WHAT NOW?

It's amazing how far we've come in the fight against cancer. New advances in science and technology bring us ever closer to unraveling the mystery of how cancer cells grow and spread. As a result, the odds that someone diagnosed today will live to a ripe old age continuously get better. Statistics from the American Cancer Society (ACS) indicate that between 1993 and 1999, the rate of cancer deaths declined by 8.4 percent in men and 3.3 percent in women.

The gains made against cancer are significant. Nonetheless, the ACS estimates that doctors will diagnose more than 1.3 million new cases of the disease in the United States by the end of 2005. In men, cancers of the prostate, lung, colon, and rectum are most common; in women, cancers of the breast, lung, colon, and rectum occur most often.

Cancer can be virulent, aggressive, and unrelenting. According to the ACS, more than 570,000 Americans will die from the disease in 2005. In other words, cancer will be responsible for one in every four deaths in the United States. This is partly because of population growth, especially among the elderly. As people live longer, their chances of getting cancer increase.

These statistics are meant not to discourage you but to provide perspective as you begin your cancer journey. Through the pages ahead, you will learn how to tap into your innate cleverness, resourcefulness, and energy to outwit cancer. You will learn how to achieve and maintain a positive attitude and dignity in the face of a deadly enemy. Perhaps most important, you will learn how to enlist the help of other people. Because although we will encourage you to find within yourself old-fashioned virtues like willpower, discipline, coolness, and courage under pressure, your cancer battle need not be a heroic, *lonely* struggle.

We want to make it clear that when we talk about "outwitting" cancer, we are not promising a cure. Even though you might not necessarily beat the disease in the end, we believe that you can still "get the better of [it] by superior ingenuity and cleverness," to borrow from Webster's definition of *outwit*. We who know cancer understand that it is a disease not only of the body but also of the mind and the spirit, where its chief symptoms are fear and a sense of isolation. When you beat them, you knock cancer to the ropes. You cannot merely survive; you must thrive throughout the entire process, from diagnosis through treatment and remission or—depending on its course—through recurrence and the end of life. You can still have the last laugh on cancer by adopting and nurturing a healthy mind-set.

This book will ask you to put your wits to work, to move into action and fight hard to win every battle, knowing you may not win the whole war. It will show you the value of believing in yourself and your support system. To outwit cancer is to believe that you *can* outwit cancer. It requires more than

strategy; it requires a conviction that you can remain hopeful in the face of your own mortality. In fact, research shows that those people who believe in something have a better chance of cure.

GOD MAY HAVE A SENSE OF HUMOR, BUT WHY AREN'T I LAUGHING?

Curing cancer is not a cut-and-dried matter of diagnosis and prognosis based on medical facts, risk/benefit ratios of various treatments, the patient's stage of cancer, and the clinician's analytical and skill level. We must take into account two other critical factors that exert considerable influence in the cancer battle. They are the patient's ability to know his priorities and values in life and the patient's capacity to be proactive in his own diagnosis and treatment. Though we rarely can be sure of a cure, with a significant level of patient involvement, we can predict better treatment results and higher quality of life, regardless of the ultimate outcome.
—Saar Porrath, MD

That my husband, Saar, died of cancer—a fairly rare and quite aggressive form of multiple myeloma called plasma cell leukemia—is the ultimate irony. Saar was a radiologist and radiation and breast oncologist, specializing in breast disease. He transformed how breast disease is treated by physicians and how women are treated as patients.

Saar was a pioneer in mammography and early invasive procedures such as radiologically guided biopsy and brachytherapy, which involves implanting radioactive "seeds" in patients with ovarian and prostate cancer. He helped develop multimodality breast diagnosis, combining mammography with ultrasound, clinical examination, and other procedures to vastly increase accuracy in detecting breast cancer. He was the father of the comprehensive diagnostic breast center, starting at Santa Monica Hospital and then opening the first freestanding center, The Woman's Breast Center, in Santa Monica.

Saar practiced in Los Angeles from the mid-1970s until the year before his death in 1999, saving the lives—and often the breasts—of thousands of women. He lectured around the world, serving on regional, national, and international boards and committees, tirelessly seeking to bring greater knowledge about breast cancer to professional and lay audiences alike.

Through all of this, Saar never lost sight of his lifelong goal of training doctors and other health care professionals to have greater sensitivity in their communication with patients. Though he could be gruff, he cared deeply about his own patients, and he let them know it. They understood that his heart was in the right place, and they valued his frank talk as much as his professional skills and guidance. Many said that he made them feel part of the process, that he encouraged them to be proactive partners in getting the best available information before making decisions about their treatment and care.

In his practice, Saar tried to be there for his patients as much as possible. He provided insight into the disease generally and their cases specifically; he passed on information about treatment options and clinical trials; he recommended physicians for consultations and second opinions; and he offered referrals to practitioners of complementary and alternative therapies. He even volunteered a sympathetic ear or a shoulder to cry on, when that's what was called for.

Saar set out to clinically validate his individualized, patient-centered approach to cancer treatment and care. If his approach held up over time and through many patients, he would codify his methodology into a system that others could follow. It was, he said, "a lofty ideal." But he knew that the key to cancer remission lay in the patient/doctor partnership.

As Saar listened to each patient's medical, psychological, and lifestyle history, he tried to discern their hopes and fears about their illnesses. He would use this information to customize his protocols for them. He kept track of what advice he gave and how he gave it, as well as what advice his patients followed and what they ignored—all toward the end of improved patient-doctor communication, improved treatment and care, and, ultimately, improved outcomes.

Saar's interactions with his patients generated the qualitative data that formed the foundation of an effective cancer management program. They also gave credibility to his theories about the value of cancer patient advocacy. He continually refined his methodology over his 25-year career in oncology. When he developed cancer, his own experiences as a patient—and mine as his personal advocate—fed into this body of knowledge. We polished our collective wisdom into a

10-step Personal Cancer Management System (PCMS), codifying and simplifying it for patients and their loved ones, adding exercises and tools that would hone the necessary skills for taking charge of cancer from the moment of diagnosis.

CANCER FROM A PATIENT'S PERSPECTIVE

You might think that as a respected oncologist, Saar would have been at an advantage in terms of his treatment and care. We learned otherwise. Though Saar could interpret his own test reports and could identify treatment options about as well as any of the physicians he dealt with, we were amazed, angered, frustrated, humiliated, and disappointed by the hurdles we encountered. We could only imagine what other patients without his "insider" status might be facing.

There were occasions when being a physician and a psychologist gave us a definite edge. We were able to access resources and experts more easily and more quickly than someone outside the system. We were on surer ground in asking for records and treatments. Once, the head nurse at an unresponsive hospital turned out to be the daughter of a patient of Saar's. Upon recognizing him, she went to great lengths to get us the information we needed. But the rest of the time, we were just another couple on the cancer conveyor belt, struggling against the machinery of the medical establishment.

As such, we realized very early in the process that we needed help. So we turned to family and friends to help pick up the slack—

shuttling Saar between his office and his twice-a-day chemotherapy sessions, running errands for us, sometimes just calling to stay in touch. Also, because the complexities of cancer prohibit even specialists from knowing everything about the disease, we decided early on to work with a team of oncologists rather than just one. All of these experts agreed to be available to us, whether in person or by conference call, at pivotal stages throughout Saar's ordeal. Such a team approach has built-in checks and balances, which is invaluable when processing so much input.

Throughout his career, Saar had been very open to complementary and alternative medicine (CAM), combining the most effective CAM therapies with the best conventional treatments in what has become known as an integrated medicine approach. So we surrounded ourselves with other health professionals who were experts in CAM disciplines—including a fitness trainer, a nutritionist, an herbalist, a massage therapist, an acupuncturist, a chiropractor, a cognitive retraining specialist (to address the cognitive and neurological effects of chemotherapy), and even a Tibetan meditation instructor (to help with stress reduction and sleep problems). We were willing to accept the wisdom of anyone from any tradition, as long as we felt it might improve Saar's health.

ADVOCACY TAKES ON NEW IMPORTANCE

Saar's illness presented an opportunity to test his theories about the value of cancer patient advocacy. He had routinely assumed the role of advocate in his practice, helping thousands of patients obtain better care, better results, and better quality of life. Many of them had beaten cancer. Now Saar was the patient, and I was his advocate.

As a psychologist, I had spent years counseling patients—including cancer patients—and serving as an executive and leadership coach and corporate consultant. As an activist, I had spoken on behalf of health care, political, feminist, and leadership causes at the local and national level. As a mother, I had loved, nurtured, and counseled my children. But my most defining personal experience was in becoming a personal advocate for the man I had loved and been married to for a quarter century. In our last few years together, he relied on me to help him through an experience that no one should face alone.

Throughout this book, we will stress the importance of recruiting a personal advocate as soon as possible after diagnosis. You need someone who can ask the right questions for you, listen and interpret for you, decipher and explain your options to you, speak with doctors and other professionals on your behalf, wrestle with the medical and insurance bureaucracies, and fight any and all battles for you. In short, this person can get you what you need—whether it's information from the Internet or a glass of water.

In Step 1 (page 1), we'll delve into the process of finding a personal advocate in much more detail. It can be a spouse or partner, a parent or child, a sibling or another family member, or a close friend. With this relationship as a foundation, reaching out and including others in your cancer journey becomes that much easier.

If you and your personal advocate encounter a particularly challenging situation, or if the two of you are struggling to make a decision, you might consider expanding your team to include a cancer patient advocate (CPA). The CPA is a primary care physician, psychiatrist, or medical psychologist who has specialized training in cancer care. He or she helps cancer patients (and families) manage the myriad issues that arise in planning for treatment and care. From this partnership, others may grow. For example, a CPA could secure referrals to a variety of cancer specialists, such as a surgical oncologist, radiation oncologist, and research medical oncologist (often a national expert in your particular kind of cancer). The CPA also can help assemble a team of CAM practitioners. The overlapping relationships among these professionals will provide as good a safety net as we humans can construct.

Senator Hillary Clinton once proclaimed, "It takes a village to raise a child." In much the same way, it takes a small corps of caring individuals to support a cancer patient. It starts with the power of two: the patient and the personal advocate.

RETHINKING CANCER TREATMENT AND CARE

Saar was a born sponge for information and a natural teacher. When he went into remission 8 months after his diagnosis, he felt he had learned so much about the cancer process—the successes and failures, the shortcuts and detours, the smart moves and not-so-smart ones—that he instinctively wanted to pass on his knowledge to others. So he began writing this book.

Now Saar could see cancer through a dual lens. His odyssey had taken him from cancer specialist to cancer patient, from medical insider to frustrated outsider, from advocate to dependent. He chose to base the book as much on our personal experience as on our professional expertise. He carefully documented both sides with honesty, humor, and absolute coolness. For my part, I've combined Saar's words with my own to reinforce the "we" aspect of the Personal Cancer Management System.

The 10 steps of the PCMS, which we present through the rest of the book, build on three core principles.

- Be proactive.

- Be inclusive.

- Get an advocate.

We've designed the steps of the system so that you, as the patient, can accumulate a great deal of information about yourself and your illness. We recommend reading the steps sequentially, completing the exercises and worksheets as you go. As you'll see, we address certain topics over several chapters. This pattern of revisiting key issues is true to life, as we've learned from our own and our patients' experience. Nevertheless, if you feel as though you've already got the gist of a particular step, feel free to skip ahead. The point of the PCMS is to get you what you need.

In short, be as proactive with this book as we encourage you to be with your illness. Don't just read it. Put it to work for you. Make it your own.

Incidentally, the three core principles of the PCMS also happen to be the philosophic core of the Porrath Foundation for Cancer Patient Advocacy, which Saar and I established. As president of the foundation, I have taken responsibility for supporting and publicizing cancer patient advocacy among cancer patients and their loved ones. The foundation also provides CPA training for primary care physicians, psychiatrists, and medical psychologists. (Psychiatrists and medical psychologists who work with cancer patients are sometimes known as psycho-oncologists.)

Through the efforts of the Porrath Foundation and other organizations, the field of cancer patient advocacy will continue to grow. You will read more about this movement throughout the book.

MORE TO GAIN THAN A CURE

Even before research confirmed it, Saar understood that laughter is good medicine. It fortifies the immune system and improves mood—both essential to fighting cancer. For Saar, humor was an all-purpose elixir, good for breaking the ice with patients and loosening the uptightness of certain peers. Not that he always told jokes. He simply had honed an ability to defuse almost any difficult situation with a little levity.

When Saar became very ill, Susie Vaughn—the massage therapist whom he had consulted during his cancer treatment—wrote this about him.

At our very first session, Saar told me that he didn't think much of massage as a therapy.

Over the course of a year and a half, he often came to my massage table in discomfort or pain, and even grouchy from all of his medications. I would attempt to cheer him by telling jokes. But Saar knew almost every one ever written. Early on, he offered me an extra $10 for any joke he hadn't heard before. I think I made an extra $20 over the year and a half!

At our last session, Saar was softer. He told me his three favorite jokes. I think they were his farewell gift to me.

But Saar's real gift was the courage he showed me every time he got up on my table, ready to just "receive" (a near impossibility for a long-time caregiver like him). His other gift was the compassion and respect he gave me, as his caregiver, when he took the time to say good-bye.

Neither Saar's famous humor nor his voracious appetite for life—nor his notorious competitive instinct, nor his towering intellectual prowess—could ward off the aggressive and unrelenting strain of cancer that eventually took his life. But that happened only after he—and I, alongside him as his personal advocate—put up an equally aggressive and unrelenting fight.

Two years after his diagnosis, Saar succumbed to cancer. But the cancer did not win. We lived our active and vital life to the end. It enabled Saar—a man not known for effusive demonstrations of affection—to show deep love for his family and friends. It motivated those around him to return that love. Certainly, it inspired the two of us to fall in love all over again.

Our fight against Saar's cancer brought us so much closer together as a couple that in some odd way, I am almost—repeat, almost—glad we went through it, despite how it ended. In the years of his illness, we came to appreciate each other even more. We touched more. We hugged more. We laughed more. We expressed our feelings for each other more. I can say, without embarrassment, that we made love more and better than at almost any other time in our 25-year marriage.

Through the process of caregiving and care-receiving over the course of Saar's diagnosis and treatment, we learned so much—about the true nature of cancer; about the ins and outs of the health care system; about the loyalty of family and close friends; about our own strengths and weaknesses, our tolerance of physical and psychological pain, our capacity for love and empathy. The lessons learned have served me well.

In the course of writing this book, I learned that I had cancer. The PCMS guided me from diagnosis to cure. I'm happy to report that I'm speaking to you as a cancer survivor. I'll share more of my story in the Epilogue (page 189). It has given me a new perspective on and appreciation for the knowledge that Saar and I present here. May it serve as guideposts for your own cancer journey.

Early in the 21st century, our sincerest wish is that by the end of it, cancer will have joined diseases like smallpox as a footnote in medical history. Then books like this one will become obsolete. Yet even with all of the advances in diagnostic and treatment techniques, cancer probably will remain with us for some time to come. Together, starting here, we can fight the disease with determination and hope.

NOW! TAKE CONTROL

"You have cancer."

Three words, four syllables from the mouth of a doctor, and suddenly you're playing by a new set of rules. You're more sensitive to your own limits and to your own mortality. You may feel as though you're living on borrowed time . . . but who's the lender?

Grand plans and ambitions no longer are important. Instead, you find new meaning in the here and now—the loved ones you spend your down-time with; the dinners and walks you enjoy; the phone calls and letters you receive.

Chances are, your old way of dealing with stress won't work anymore. You can't just "tough things out." And getting angry will drain your energy, which you can't afford. You need to stay strong to fight your illness.

You may feel as though your personal affairs have become everyone else's business. By the same token, you may feel less isolated and alone than before.

You have much to learn and much to adapt to. But this battle is *your* battle. Now is the time to assert control over your life, over your body and your emotions.

With a disease like cancer, of course, some things are beyond your control. We realize that. What we're suggesting is that you take control of what you can. In fact, giving up the illusion of total control is an important first step toward planning and executing realistic strategies. From the start, you know that you'll win some and you'll lose some, but you'll always fight the good fight.

Perhaps not surprisingly, taking control is the first step in the Personal Cancer Management System (PCMS), which my husband, Saar, created and I contributed to, and which has continued to evolve with time and use. The PCMS consists of 10 steps, each of which builds on Saar's and my collective experiences with thousands of patients, as well as with Saar's own illness.

The foundation of the PCMS consists of three principles that also are essential to taking control.

- Be proactive.
- Be inclusive.
- Get an advocate.

By learning and applying these principles from the beginning of the cancer process, you will stick with them all the way through. All three require you to take action, to do what you know is necessary to manage and ultimately defeat your illness. All three require you to involve others—some whom you already know, others whom you haven't yet met.

In troubled times, many of us want to be alone, to isolate ourselves from others. You need to overcome that impulse. By allowing others to shoulder some of the burden, you can concentrate on the single most important task before you: getting well.

BE PROACTIVE

From others' research, as well as our own, we know that those cancer patients who are the most proactive achieve better results and a better quality of life. *Proactive* is a relatively new term. You might hear it in the context of describing someone who takes charge of a situation or who otherwise acts in a positive or preemptive manner. By definition, it means "acting in anticipation of future problems, needs, or changes." It means not merely thinking but using forethought.

Being proactive is the opposite of being passive, of seeing yourself as the victim. It is about outsmarting forces that may be working against you. It involves taking action rather than sitting back and waiting for something to happen or for someone to tell you what to do. It requires asking questions, contemplating the answers, and using them to formulate a plan of action. It's about taking charge of your disease and treatment, your health and recovery, your *life*.

Being proactive does not guarantee that if you look long enough and hard enough, you'll discover a magic bullet—a cure. Cancer treatment is about mostly small triumphs, not one big breakthrough victory.

To explain, big victories can be few and far between. If you put all of your energy into them and they don't materialize, optimism and hope will give way to anxiety and agitation. They trigger the release of norepinephrine and cortisol, "stress hormones" that in turn weaken your immune system. Now more than ever, your immune system—your body's first line of defense against disease—needs to be at its best.

Small triumphs, on the other hand, are more attainable. They create a sense of achievement, which translates to longer upbeat stretches and less chronic stress. In this way, they help maintain a healthy immune function.

PCMS Tool #1.1: Consider Quality of Life

Among the key elements of being proactive is having a voice in your own treatment. In his practice, Saar noticed that those patients who were most likely to beat cancer were the ones who collaborated with their doctors in making decisions about treatment programs and posttreatment rehabilitation. In general, they were more receptive and cooperative and less stressed-out than patients who simply followed their doctors' orders.

Even for Saar, who was a teacher as well as a doctor, this power of patients to improve their own outcomes was a surprise. He made even more of an effort to include his patients in thinking about the disease. He encouraged them to view their relationships with him as partnerships. It was good for them. He continually refined this methodology over his 25 years in oncology. When he became ill, he formed partnerships with those who administered his treatment or assisted in it in some way.

In today's cost-conscious health care system, where doctor-patient face time can be all too brief, being proactive has become partic-

ularly important. It allows you to get the most from each appointment. Throughout this book, we'll provide the necessary tools for collecting and evaluating information, so you're able to make informed decisions about all aspects of your treatment. Among the most indispensable of these tools is your cancer notebook, which you'll begin compiling in Step 3 (page 57).

Before we immerse ourselves in those details, though, we need to spend some time on quality of life, which comes up often in this book. As you'll see, it plays a vital role in the decision-making process.

In the weeks and months ahead, you probably will be getting a lot of advice from other people—people who are basing their opinions on what *they* expect and value. They may insist that you continue treatment even though it's too debilitating for you or that you give up when you're ready to soldier on. What they'll tell you is valid—*for them.* You have no obligation to take their advice to heart. Smile politely . . . and ignore them.

To determine what quality of life means to you personally, ask yourself the following questions.

- Do I need to continue working to feel as though I'm a contributing member of society?

- Do I need to be a major player for my friends to want to spend time with me? Can I maintain my present level of activity?

- Suppose I choose to spend my time reading, talking with my spouse (or children or grandchildren), or listening

Joan's Triumph

Joan came to see me a few months after she had been diagnosed with pancreatic cancer. Fortunately, the illness had been discovered at an early stage. This made Joan eligible for the Whipple procedure, a surgical intervention that offers patients with pancreatic cancer their best chance at remission. Joan decided to undergo the 11-hour surgery; when it was successful, she was elated. Immediately afterward, she started chemotherapy.

The first protocol did not effectively contain Joan's disease. She changed medications and subsequently developed complications. Then an infection made her very sick, hospitalizing her for several weeks.

Joan told me that when the surgery was successful, she assumed that the chemotherapy would just be insurance. When that turned out to be untrue, her spirits took a nosedive.

As we talked, Joan revealed another issue that undoubtedly was taking a psychological toll. Her father had died from pancreatic cancer after a long battle. As Joan went from doctor to doctor, consultation to consultation, she could not erase from her mind the thought that she was bound to come to the same end as her father—a man whom she had always been told she took after.

Even after Joan recovered from her infection and resumed chemotherapy, depression hung over her like a dark cloud. This time her tumors were shrinking, yet she remained despondent, eventually becoming more and more isolated. "Why should I try anything?" she asked me. "It's all a pipe dream. It gets you in the end anyway. It got my dad, didn't it?"

I couldn't promise a happy ending, but I knew that Joan wasn't focused on her own condition. She was reliving the death

to my favorite CD. Will I feel that I'm boring?

- I may be in pain, or I may have trouble with treatment or its side effects. What will keep me going through the discomfort?

- What makes life worth living?

Your answers to the first three questions should shed some light on what defines your self-esteem and self-worth, which color your quality of life. Your job, your relationships, and your interests and activities help shape your identity as a person. For example, suppose you're at a social event and someone asks what you do for a living, why you stopped volunteering at the local food bank, or whether you've played golf lately. Even though you're fighting cancer, your response might take on an awkward or apologetic tone.

of her father, and this distraction weakened her. She slept and ate badly, which robbed her of vital energy.

Realistically, their situations were not as similar as Joan thought. Her father had died 20 years earlier; medical science had come a long way since then. Just as important, her illness had been caught earlier. Yet Joan refused to see the importance of these distinctions. A more positive outlook on her treatment, and her life, surely could make a dramatic difference.

As I looked at Joan, I felt as though her father were in the room with us. So I brought him into the conversation. I reminded her of his bravery. "Would your dad want you to give up the fight?" I asked her. I reminded her of the stories she had proudly told me of his repeated attempts to beat the disease. I got her to focus on the idea of short-term goals, which apparently had kept her father going. I also helped her to see that emulating her father's behavior did not necessarily mean she would meet with the same fate.

Joan slowly let go of her fear of long-term failure so that she could concentrate on small victories that might eventually lead to success. She learned to enjoy the moments of hope, knowing that they would cushion the disappointment if the next rounds of treatment were less successful. She was grateful for a good night's sleep, a day without nausea, energy for errands, lunch with a friend.

Joan realized that while control of the big picture might be beyond her reach, control of the small picture was not. She could make improvements in her quality of life that would ease her depression and anxiety—and that, in turn, might lead to better treatment outcomes. Seeing her illness from this new perspective helped lift her out of despair.

On some level, you feel like less of a person.

The remaining two questions reveal your thoughts about treatment, including how hard and how long you're willing to keep fighting. For example, the side effects of chemotherapy or radiation may become so intolerable that you choose to stop treatment. Or perhaps you will choose to try an unconventional therapy over a more aggressive cancer protocol. To some degree, quality of life will set the course for your care.

As you ponder these questions and your answers, consider how your relationship with your doctor might factor in. If the two of you are able to exchange information and ideas in a way that gives you a sense of control over your treatment, it can have a positive effect on your quality of life. Such uninhibited interaction is central to a true doctor-patient partnership.

PCMS Tool #1.2: Determine Your Information-Gathering Style

Being proactive also involves educating yourself about your particular kind of cancer and your options for treatment. As you gather information, you'll feel more in control of your disease—that is, as long as you don't amass more data than you can digest.

Information is like the flotsam in a shipwreck. Don't insist on searching for the lifeboat when a life preserver will do. Determine what you need for now, and move forward from there.

All of us have unique information-gathering styles; we require varying amounts and types of data to make decisions. It's important to know your own style so that you're not frustrated by having too little information or swamped by having too much.

Which sort of information gatherer are you? Read the following two descriptions and place a check next to the one that best describes you.

☐ *High-information intellects* need to know everything about a situation in order to make a decision. They're confident that they can reach the right decision with all of the facts. They also want to be in control and are uncomfortable giving away authority. For cancer patients, time and energy are limited, so their sense of control and authority will be challenged.

☐ *Low-information intuitives* are able to make decisions with a "good enough" level of facts. They're more likely to act on hunches, and they prefer to delegate control rather than using up energy fretting over a particular decision. They're comfortable putting themselves in the hands of an expert. They have an easier time asking for help—something every cancer patient must do.

Once you've identified your information-gathering style, start thinking about the sort of information you want to find. As mentioned above, your time and energy are limited, so you should use your resources wisely. Ignore those scenes from old movies in which doctors work night after sleepless night searching for an answer. Switch off the tape in your head that says, "When you want a job done right, do it yourself." Ask someone to help with your research. By assigning this task to another person, you'll be able to zero in on precisely what you're looking for. You'll need to, so you can give clear instructions and get what you want.

Through this process, pay attention to how much stress you're feeling. Stress is a good barometer. When you have more information than you can absorb, you'll feel overwhelmed. When you have too little, you'll feel helpless. Your goal is to be comfortable.

PCMS Tool #1.3: Work SMART

Whether you're a high-information intellect or a low-information intuitive, the key to effective information gathering is working smarter, not harder. In fact, we suggest using SMART as a guide for your search. SMART is an acronym that stands for *s*pecific, *m*easurable, *a*chievable, *r*ealistic, and *t*ime-bound. SMART answers always have these five elements.

For example, let's say that you need information on lymphoma. Here's how SMART might shape your search.

- *Specific:* Depending on your preference and expertise, tap your available resources—your doctor, the Internet, or your local library—to find the following types of information: (1) articles by nationally known lymphoma experts, (2) available clinical trials for lymphoma patients, (3) survivor groups, and (4) books on coping with cancer.

- *Measurable:* Aim for three examples of each of the types of information above.

- *Achievable:* Limit your search to what you can easily obtain through your resources.

- *Realistic:* Make sure you have the support you need to get the information you're looking for. For example, if you're not comfortable using the Internet, ask for help from a family member or friend who's more tech-savvy. Online search services also are available for a fee.

- *Time-bound:* Set a date for completing your search.

As you move forward with the PCMS, you'll find that the SMART model can come in handy for all kinds of searches—from finding an oncologist who specializes in your kind of cancer to exploring complementary and alternative therapies for managing pain. It helps narrow the field of information, while delivering the necessary level of detail to make sound decisions.

PCMS Tool #1.4: Find Health Information on the Internet

Throughout this book, you'll see references to Web sites that Saar and I found particularly reliable and useful, whether through our patients' experiences or our own. The Internet is a marvelous tool for being proactive. We're fortunate to live in an age when an entire world of knowledge and expertise is as close as a click of a button. But if you've spent any time online, you know that all that information can be a bit too much to digest. Simply entering the word *cancer*, or even a specific kind of cancer, in a search engine can turn up thousands of Web sites.

Applying the SMART model will help you sort through all the data. So, too, will asking the right questions. Continuing with lymphoma as an example, you can narrow your search from the start by determining what you need to know. You can do that by asking the following:

- Do I want more information than I'm able to gather from books and magazines?

- What hasn't my doctor told me about lymphoma?

- Am I looking for a general overview, a list of facts and statistics, or a more in-depth explanation?

- Do I need help deciphering medical terminology?

- Do I want to read about the very latest advances in lymphoma research, including experimental treatments?

- Who are the top lymphoma experts? Where do I find them?

Once you determine the answers to these questions, you can use them to map out your online search. But where should you look first?

Your best bet is to start with the megasites below. They offer many levels of information, including overviews, statistics, access to the latest research developments, descriptions of clinical trials, and links to other resources such as medical journals and support groups. The home page for each site has a search option, where you can type in what you're looking for.

- Abramson Cancer Center of the University of Pennsylvania: oncolink.upenn.edu

- American Cancer Society: www.cancer.org

- Cancer*Care:* www.cancercare.org

- National Cancer Institute: www.cancer.gov

- New York Online Access to Health: www.noah-health.org (click on "Health Topics," then "Cancer")

- The Wellness Community: www.thewellnesscommunity.org

For a comprehensive list of community cancer centers by state, check out this site:

- Association of Community Cancer Centers: www.accc-cancer.org (click on "Find a Cancer Center")

If you're interested in news from the front line of cancer research, try the following:

- The health sections of most major newspapers—e.g., the *New York Times:* www.nytimes.com (under "News," click on "Health")

For basic information such as dictionaries, directories, and drug profiles, try:

- Healthfinder: www.healthfinder.gov

- MedlinePlus: www.medlineplus.gov

We're not suggesting that you visit all of these Web sites in one sitting—although if that's your style, feel free. You need to find the right balance between gathering information, or being proactive, and managing stress. Remember, you can always recruit someone else to do the searching for you, if you're finding the sites too much to sort through. *Doable* and *comfortable* should be your mantras now.

To learn more about conducting effective online searches, see Resources (page 193), or visit the Porrath Foundation for Cancer Patient Advocacy Web site: www.porrath foundation.org.

BE INCLUSIVE

Being inclusive means, simply, letting others in. It correlates with Saar's original observation that cancer patients who formed partnerships with their doctors had the best chance of survival.

These patients were proactive about their partnerships. They brought information to their appointments and asked many questions about it. They didn't hesitate to express differences of opinion when planning their treatments. They sought out second opinions as

Shelly's Refusal

Shelly was one of Saar's celebrity patients. On film, she was one of the most dynamic and charismatic performers in the business. Perhaps not surprisingly, she was ferociously private when the cameras stopped rolling. She also was accustomed to having things her way. In fact, she demanded it. Her determination, as much as her talent, had gotten her where she wanted to go.

When Saar told Shelly she had breast cancer, she set about fighting it with a vengeance. "I'll beat this thing," she announced. "And like everything else in my life, I'll beat it alone." When she went into remission, she assumed she had dodged the cancer bullet. It was another in a long series of personal achievements.

Shelly was faithful about her posttreatment checkups. Nonetheless, 10 years later, tests revealed cancer in her cervix. She reacted differently this time around. At first, she sank into a deep depression. She delayed treatment. When she finally acquiesced, she found the situation abhorrent. She withdrew to her room, climbed into bed, and literally pulled the covers over her head.

Those closest to Shelly were upset, baffled, and frustrated by her behavior. They encouraged her to fight the good fight as she had so often before. Their attempts to help made her angry. Now she refused to fight with the same determination that had made her successful.

When the cancer spread and began to take its toll, Shelly's family wanted to spend time with her, if only to share her precious last days. She pushed them away. Beyond family, she had friends; beyond that, a support group of millions. She chose not to draw on any of them.

Then and now, those closest to Shelly feel that her last days could have been better. Saar believed that had she let her family in, let them help her, she might have lived longer—and if not longer, certainly with more joy in her final days.

---

well as complementary and alternative therapies—and they told their doctors about it.

When you open up to another person—whether a doctor, a family member, or a friend—in this way, you lift some of the burden from your own shoulders, so you don't exhaust yourself physically or psychologically. A large and growing body of medical research confirms that our physical and psychological health improves when we reach out to others. Poets and songwriters have been telling us the same thing forever: "No man is an island, no man stands alone"; "That's what friends are for"; "Lean on me."

Reaching out to others is an innate human response. All of us have seen what happens when a child falls and skins her knee. Afraid and hurting, she'll look around for someone to comfort her and maybe stop the pain. If she doesn't see a familiar face, she might even settle for a stranger. Unfortunately, as we grow up, we're taught to "be brave" by keeping our feelings—and our need for support and solace—to ourselves.

If you're in an early stage of cancer, you may feel strong and able to handle most tasks on your own. Odds are, that will change in the weeks and months ahead. You may not feel terrible physically, but your illness will make demands on your time and energy. Your life was hectic before your diagnosis. Now you must make room in your schedule for doctors' appointments, diagnostic tests, and treatments. You may need to adjust your work hours or find new arrangements for child care. You may spend hours on the phone navigating the red tape of insurance claims. You don't want to throw up your hands and give in. But you can see how having someone to lend a hand—or an ear to listen or a shoulder to lean on—could make a huge difference.

Of course, some people are very private by nature. Perhaps you're reluctant to open up about something as personal as a cancer diagnosis, or you don't want to "burden" others with your illness. Why not let those people decide for themselves? Think about how good you feel when you're able to reach out and help someone. Now is your opportunity to let someone else share in that same experience. Don't let modesty or bravery stand in the way of such transformative chemistry.

Even if you have been a loner all of your life, you need to realize that you're in a situation that you may not be able to get through all by yourself. At the very least, reaching out to others allows you to put more of your energy into healing. As noted historian Studs Terkel once said, "Take it easy, but take it." By letting go, you actually gain control—over your cancer, and your life.

PCMS Tool #1.5: Acknowledge Your Reluctance to Need Others

Being inclusive is a conscious decision. You must choose to share. For some people, this can be very difficult. It means leaving one's shell and revealing many emotions and needs.

Reaching out to others means facing issues that you may find uncomfortable. What stands in your way is a knot of habits, beliefs, and fears known as resistors, which conspire to isolate you from those around you.

Below is a list of emotional responses that can create inclusiveness when you share them with someone else. Check the ones that you wouldn't feel comfortable confiding to another person.

☐ I need help, but I'm reluctant to ask for it.

☐ I want to reach out to others, but I feel embarrassed or guilty.

☐ Sometimes I feel scared.

☐ I see my life as valuable.

☐ I know that I'm loved.

If you checked even one of the above statements, the exercises ahead should be especially helpful for you. We hope that you'll do them regardless of your "score," as they present principles and techniques that you'll be using throughout this book.

Barriers to Asking for Help

We humans are creatures of habit, with set patterns of thoughts, emotions, and behaviors. If we change our lives, it's because we're driven by a crisis or some other intense experience, and we use it as a wake-up call. Cancer is such an experience.

Often our first reaction to adjusting our set patterns is negative. This is especially true in the context of becoming more inclusive. You might interpret your desire to reach out to others as weakness; you might feel embarrassed by asking for help, ashamed by even needing to do so. These are legitimate reactions, rooted in a pattern of avoiding dependence on others. Perhaps you fear rejection; perhaps you worry about coming across as selfish or demanding or stupid. You may not want to let on that you feel vulnerable.

These reactions are *resistors*—barriers to asking for help. They tend to hide beneath the surface, bubbling up when you least expect them. For example, you put off phoning a friend because you get a knot in your stomach each time you reach for the receiver. Then when you finally make the call, you talk about everything except what's most important: asking for help.

You may realize that you're avoiding the inevitable, but you can't seem to help yourself. Resistors are known for provoking procrastination. When you keep putting off a task, you're avoiding an opportunity that eventually could save your life.

Resistors may kick in as a consequence of the actions of others. Certain cues set them off. Those cues are *triggers*. Think of them as resistors in infant form.

A trigger may be a comment like "I'm busy; can we talk later?" You may interpret that as "Don't bother me; I'm not interested in you." But chances are, the person meant just what he said—nothing more, nothing less.

Old beliefs can enable us to rationalize our resistors and triggers. For example, most of us were raised to view doctors as authority figures. We may feel perfectly comfortable asking questions and sharing information with them under normal circumstances. But that changes when a serious illness such as cancer enters the picture. Then we subconsciously revert to that image of the all-knowing doctor, with ourselves as the obedient children.

We must recognize this as an old, obsolete belief and push ourselves past it in order to form meaningful, productive partnerships with our doctors. As adults, we should see our doctors as peers with whom we can have meaningful dialogue, learning from their medical expertise and making decisions based on mutual input and discourse.

Take a moment to read through the following lists. Do any of the reactions and resistors seem familiar to you? If so, take heart: They're here because they're quite common. You may want to refer back to these lists as you complete the next four exercises.

Sample Tasks

- Accompany me to doctor's appointments.

- Drive to treatments.

- Chauffeur the kids to after-school activities.

- Shop for groceries.
- Help with insurance paperwork.
- Go out to lunch or a movie.

Possible Reactions

- I feel stupid asking someone to do this for me.
- This is ridiculous.
- I feel like a child.
- Why must I do this?
- I'm totally embarrassed.
- What a dumb idea.
- This is so unnecessary.
- They won't have time for this.
- They wouldn't want to commit to doing this.
- I don't have time to find someone to help me.

Possible Resistors

- Denial
- Embarrassment or shame
- Anger, sometimes expressed as irritation or frustration
- Procrastination
- Shyness
- Self-righteousness ("If I want something done right, I'll do it myself")
- Need to please
- Need to be in control
- Helplessness
- A Pollyanna attitude ("Everything's fine")
- Fear of dependency

PCMS Tool #1.6: Assess Your Willingness to Be Inclusive

This exercise can help identify possible resistors that may be undermining your efforts to seek help from others. In the first column of the worksheet, make a list of 10 tasks with which you could use assistance. Break down each task into specific, actionable steps, and write these in the second column. Use the third column to rate each task according to the following scale.

1 = Hard to ask for and do

2 = Less hard to ask for and do

3 = Easy to ask for and do

In the last column, make note of any resistors that may be keeping you from carrying out the tasks you jotted down. (If you need help, refer to the list at left, as well as the sample worksheet.)

Once you've filled in all four columns, add up your ratings. If your total score is between 10 and 17, you probably are very resistant to reaching out to others, and you will need to work at becoming inclusive. If it's between 18 and 24, you're somewhat resistant; 25 or higher, you likely are very sociable and comfortable asking for help.

PCMS Tool #1.7: Identify Your Resistors

Now that you've zeroed in on possible resistors, you can use the exercise on page 16 to understand how they're interfering with your ability to ask for the help you need. You can see patterns in the resistors and in the triggers that are set off by certain people, places, and situations.

PCMS Tool #1.6 (Sample)

HOW INCLUSIVE ARE YOU? A Self-Assessment

TASKS	NECESSARY STEPS	DIFFICULTY RATING	POSSIBLE RESISTORS
1. Schedule a walking partner three days per week.	Call: __Pat __John __Kate	2	I am afraid they won't want to spend so much time with me—embarrassment, shyness, fear of rejection.
2. Get a second opinion.	Ask Tracy to help write a script so that I can practice asking my oncologist for a referral.	2	I am too tired—embarrassment, anger at needing people.

PCMS Tool #1.6

HOW INCLUSIVE ARE YOU? A Self-Assessment

TASKS	NECESSARY STEPS	DIFFICULTY RATING	POSSIBLE RESISTORS
1.			
2.			
3.			
4.			
5.			
6.			
7.			
8.			
9.			
10.			

Total _____

By identifying these patterns now, you'll be able to recognize and respond to them as you move through the steps of the PCMS.

This is a brainstorming exercise, designed to open your mind to new thinking. Brainstorming effectively means writing as fast as you can without being self-critical. In the top box, jot down what you perceive as your primary barrier to being inclusive. (Refer to the sample worksheet on the opposite page as you need to.) Then keep going until you fill in all four response boxes (A through D) and all three "Whys" in each box. Don't stop to edit your thoughts.

PCMS Tool #1.8: Take Control of Your Resistors

You may see yourself as having a unique set of complex resistors. In fact, you may define your personality in terms of what you won't do. But in our experience, resistors form rather simple patterns of thought and behavior.

Take a look at your responses in the previous exercise. You probably can pick out a pattern to your responses and the old beliefs that are driving them. They represent your most powerful and persistent resistors.

In the sample exercise, the resistors center around embarrassment, guilt, and shame. These are real feelings. But they also can be resistors to moving forward.

Using your responses in the previous exercise, fill in the worksheet on page 18. At the end, you'll come up with an action step for overcoming your resistors to being inclusive. One helpful tool is Stop! Reflect! Clarify! (SRC), which we'll discuss next.

PCMS Tool #1.9: Stop! Reflect! Clarify!

You can use the SRC exercise on page 21 to work through any resistors and triggers that are keeping you from being inclusive—as well as other challenges that arise through the cancer process. The purpose of the exercise is to help you take control of thoughts, feelings, and behaviors that aren't serving you well at this time. The three commands—Stop! Reflect! Clarify!—calm you, so you can focus on the task at hand and take action. In practice, they become a useful mantra.

For the sample exercise on page 20, we've chosen to focus on embarrassment. It's a common theme among those who feel uncomfortable asking for help. Any of the following can bring on the familiar flush of embarrassment when you're reaching out to someone.

- Becoming the center of attention
- Acknowledging that you're out of work
- Revealing that you have an imperfect body
- Suspecting that you did something "wrong" to cause your illness
- Feeling that you weren't smart enough to outwit cancer in the first place
- Admitting that you aren't strong enough to do everything for yourself
- Worrying that you will be rejected or that your request for help will be refused

Asking others for help shouldn't be a source of embarrassment, but it is—for a lot of people. Who knows why? We do know that it's a natural response, and it can be overcome.

BEING INCLUSIVE Identify Your Resistors

WHAT IS THE PROBLEM? *I can't ask my friends for help.*

A. ONE REASON IS . . .

I feel embarrassed that I can't handle everything myself.

WHY

It's my own fault for not taking better care of my health.

WHY

My mother said, "Laugh, and the world laughs with you. Cry, and you cry alone."

B. ANOTHER REASON IS . . .

I have to tell my boss soon, because I need time off for treatment. I'm afraid he'll fire me when he finds out.

WHY

My friends will turn away from me in disgust because I'm so needy.

WHY

Everybody will think I'm a wimp.

C. ANOTHER REASON IS . . .

WHY

It feels so hard to put the whole support thing together.

WHY

I might not even need help. Then I would feel stupid for asking.

WHY

This is silly. I'll figure it out on my own.

D. ANOTHER REASON IS . . .

WHY

Being the center of attention is uncomfortable.

WHY

The kids will have such a hard time with all these different people doing everything.

WHY

Maybe John can take off a few weeks, and that will solve everything. Who am I kidding? We haven't won the lottery.

BEING INCLUSIVE Identify Your Resistors

WHAT IS THE PROBLEM? _____

_____

A. ONE REASON IS . . .	B. ANOTHER REASON IS . . .
WHY	WHY
WHY	WHY
WHY	WHY
C. ANOTHER REASON IS . . .	D. ANOTHER REASON IS . . .
WHY	WHY
WHY	WHY
WHY	WHY

BEING INCLUSIVE Take Control of Your Resistors

THE ANSWERS (WHYS) THAT REPEAT ACROSS SEVERAL RESPONSES ARE:

I feel embarrassed that I can't handle everything myself.

"Laugh, and the world laughs with you. Cry, and you cry alone."

I feel stupid asking for help on simple things.

My friends will turn away from me in disgust because I'm so needy.

DO YOU SEE A PATTERN IN YOUR ANSWERS? DESCRIBE IT HERE.

I feel embarrassed and ashamed of having needs and am convinced that people will shun me when they find out.

I will be alone and rejected for being needy.

I feel so naked and exposed when I'm needy. It embarrasses me.

I feel stupid when I must ask for help.

DO YOU SEE RESISTORS IN THIS PATTERN? WHAT ARE THEY?

I've always presented such a capable, self-sufficient image that I'm embarrassed to ask for help.

It blows my image.

It makes me feel so needy to ask others to do for me. They will think I'm helpless.

OLD BELIEF:

I know it sounds silly, but I learned to believe that when you laugh, the world laughs with you. Cry, and you cry alone.

WHAT TRIGGERS ARE BEHIND THESE RESISTORS?

Now that I must face depending on others daily, I hear a tape playing in my head all the time. It feeds my embarrassment, which makes me feel stuck when it comes to asking for help. If I can let go of the outdated belief that's stopping me from doing what I need to do, I might get around this wall of embarrassment and reach out to others.

WHAT TO DO?

I'll use the SRC exercise to overcome these resistors and triggers.

BEING INCLUSIVE Take Control of Your Resistors

THE ANSWERS (WHYS) THAT REPEAT ACROSS SEVERAL RESPONSES ARE:

DO YOU SEE A PATTERN IN YOUR ANSWERS? DESCRIBE IT HERE.

DO YOU SEE RESISTORS IN THIS PATTERN? WHAT ARE THEY?

OLD BELIEF:

WHAT TRIGGERS ARE BEHIND THESE RESISTORS?

WHAT TO DO?

Get an Advocate

From the moment you learn that you have cancer, you're up against three things.

- The illness itself
- The internal resistors or obstacles that we've been talking about
- The inertia of the medical/pharmaceutical/social service systems

Of these, the illness is what you must show up for. It's what you need to focus on. It requires you to answer some tough questions, such as the following:

- How do I reconcile the conflicting opinions of doctors?
- What treatment should I choose?
- Will this treatment save my life? How much time will it buy me?
- What are the side effects?
- Are the side effects and expected outcomes consistent with the quality of life I want?
- How far is the treatment center from my home, my family, my friends? How will I get there?
- How much will treatment cost? Will insurance pay for it?
- Can I work during treatment?

We've talked briefly about how to go about collecting information. But using this data to make decisions—and then putting your decisions into action—may seem immensely difficult at times. If you're like most cancer patients, you will have days when the inertia of the medical establishment may seem as insurmountable as your illness. As always, Saar had a story to help illustrate this point.

An elderly woman made a telephone call. "Hello, Mount Sinai Hospital? I am trying to get some information on a patient at your hospital—I mean, all the information, not just if she's doing okay, but everything. Could you connect me with someone who could help me?"

The receptionist replied, "That's a very unusual request. Would you please hold the line?" Then an authoritative voice came on. "Are you the lady calling to get information about a patient here?" the doctor asked.

"Yes, darling," she said. "Can you tell me about Sara Franklin in Room 302?"

"Franklin, Franklin," he said, looking through his charts. "Yes, here, Franklin. Mrs. Franklin is doing very well. Her blood pressure is fine. Her blood work just came back—normal. The heart monitor will come off this afternoon. Her appetite is good, and she's doing well with physical therapy. If things continue like this, I'm sure we'll be able to release her by noon Thursday."

"Noon Thursday?" the woman nearly shouted. "Thank God. That's wonderful news. I'm so happy. Fantastic."

"I gather you must be a close family member or best friend of the patient?" the doctor asked.

"What family? What friend? I'm Sara Franklin. My doctor tells me nothing."

It's a funny story, but it illustrates a sad truth about patient/doctor communication in today's health care system. The politics of

(continued on page 22)

19

BEING INCLUSIVE Stop! Reflect! Clarify!

MY GOAL

Overcome embarrassment about asking for help.

STOP! REFLECT ON THESE QUESTIONS

WHAT AM I DOING RIGHT NOW TO PREVENT MYSELF FROM GETTING WHAT I WANT?

Ruminating about all the humiliating things I'll feel if I ask for help.

WHAT AM I FEELING RIGHT NOW?

Cringing.

HOW AM I BREATHING RIGHT NOW?

Too fast.

WHAT AM I THINKING RIGHT NOW?

I'll do it tomorrow.

WHAT TRIGGERED THESE THOUGHTS AND FEELINGS?

Giving up my "strong one" identity and admitting I need a lot of help.

CLARIFY FOR INSIGHT

WHAT IS THE REAL ISSUE?

I need my support team to help me.

WHERE DO I STAND?

Stuck.

WHAT DO I WANT TO ACCOMPLISH RIGHT NOW?

Make those calls and build a support team.

WHAT DO I WANT TO CHANGE?

Breathe slowly. Clear my mind of fears. Get unstuck.

TAKE ACTION

☑ Move toward my goal. *I choose to force myself to make the calls.*

☐ Move away from my goal.

☐ Try a new angle to reach my goal.

☐ Change my focus.

BEING INCLUSIVE Stop! Reflect! Clarify!

MY GOAL

_____

STOP! REFLECT ON THESE QUESTIONS

WHAT AM I DOING RIGHT NOW TO PREVENT MYSELF FROM GETTING WHAT I WANT?

_____

WHAT AM I FEELING RIGHT NOW?

_____

HOW AM I BREATHING RIGHT NOW?

_____

WHAT AM I THINKING RIGHT NOW?

_____

WHAT TRIGGERED THESE THOUGHTS AND FEELINGS?

_____

CLARIFY FOR INSIGHT

WHAT IS THE REAL ISSUE?

_____

WHERE DO I STAND?

_____

WHAT DO I WANT TO ACCOMPLISH RIGHT NOW?

_____

WHAT DO I WANT TO CHANGE?

_____

TAKE ACTION

☐ Move toward my goal. _____

☐ Move away from my goal. _____

☐ Try a new angle to reach my goal. _____

☐ Change my focus. _____

health care is something to take on after you're in long-term remission. Our point here is that you shouldn't depend on your doctor—or your insurance agent—to stay on top of the details of your case. Moreover, you should start planning now for the services and support that you may require down the road and probably will need to seek out on your own.

What Patients Want, What Patients Get

The Porrath Foundation conducted a survey of cancer patients and survivors, caregivers, and service providers (including oncologists, oncology nurses, hospital administrators, and cancer support organizations) in order to find out what is missing in cancer treatment. The following responses were almost universal.

- Patients needed guidance when choosing an oncologist.

- Patients found that understanding treatment options was difficult and overwhelming.

- Service providers felt that patients needed more time to explore options.

- Patients felt pressured to start treatment quickly, even without getting a second opinion.

- Patients wanted a coordinated action plan but were unsure how to go about getting one.

- Patients and those close to them agreed that many group support programs are available. But most also wanted one-on-

one counseling to sort through information and get answers about doctors, treatments, and lifestyle matters. Many also wanted personal assistance to deal with depression and other psychological issues that can follow a cancer diagnosis. Individual counseling, they said, was unavailable or difficult to come by.

As our survey showed, the network of cancer services clearly needed to close some gaps in helping cancer patients effectively manage their treatment and care. So the foundation launched a follow-up survey of service providers. From their responses, we realized that different professionals offer different kinds and levels of support. For example:

- *Oncologists and oncology nurses* won't initiate conversations about a patient's treatment. It's not that they don't care; rather, it's how they're trained. If a patient asks a specific question, the doctor or nurse will attempt to answer or may refer the patient to another specialist, such as a dietitian or psychologist.

- *Hospital administrators* are available to address questions about cancer management. But like the primary cancer care providers—the oncologists and oncology nurses—they wait for the patient to initiate the dialogue.

- *Cancer support organizations* are more proactive, especially in the area of educating cancer patients. Most offer a wide range of resources and services for the full spectrum of cancer care, from prevention and early detection to treatment and financial assistance. The options may vary considerably from one community to the next. Unfortunately, many patients have difficulty sifting through the wealth of information without assistance and guidance.

Throughout this chapter, we've talked about the importance of forming a partnership with your doctor. Indeed, a good relationship with a communicative doctor is the best one that you can have. In today's managed care environment, though, you can't count on your doctor to know and remember the minutest details of your case. Likewise, your doctor may not have time to stay abreast of advances in cancer treatment and care, which are mushrooming with the increasingly rapid pace of cancer research. You need to find someone who can focus attention on your illness and your cure. That's where the personal advocate and cancer patient advocate can pitch in.

The Personal Advocate: The Power of Two

Every cancer patient should have a personal advocate. This is the person who's there with you and for you from day one. Most likely it is a loved one to whom you already turn for help in difficult situations. It could be your spouse or partner, a brother or sister, a son or daughter, or your best friend.

The personal advocate's primary task is to be an extra set of eyes and ears, paying attention to what you cannot concentrate on. This person also provides an additional voice when you're struggling to speak on your own behalf.

The personal advocate must be willing to invest the time, energy, and emotional resources to represent your best interests in obtaining the best possible cancer treatment. It's a big responsibility, requiring a person with special skills and persistence. If your spouse or best friend travels frequently, isn't the caregiver type, or is reluctant to step into conflict or express differences of opinion, then he or she may not be the right person for the job.

The personal advocate should be someone whose thinking meshes with yours. The two of you may not agree on everything, but this person's viewpoints should challenge and intrigue you. One way or another, the two of you should synchronize. You need someone with whom you feel comfortable sharing thoughts and feelings, someone who can dispassionately analyze information and suggest a sound, sensible course of action. It won't hurt if the two of you can make each other laugh from time to time.

Your personal advocate also should demonstrate the following qualities.

- Good communication skills, both listening and speaking
- A willingness to learn medical terminology
- Empathy
- Diplomacy
- Resourcefulness
- An ability to ask difficult questions
- Discipline to not take no for an answer
- Flexibility to make time for you
- Commitment to helping you

Brooke was a bright, articulate Ivy League graduate who successfully juggled marriage, motherhood, and a successful career as a product development executive in the food industry. She was the kind of person who seemed to have planned for every contingency.

I had met Brooke a couple of years earlier, when she came to me for executive coaching to help make the transition from "mommy track" back to the fast track. Growing up in an ambitious family, she was reluctant to depend on anyone but herself. Unfortunately, this had left her intolerant of anyone else's needs. Despite that, we developed a good rapport. She broke through her issues of reluctance and intolerance, and her career once again began to thrive.

Brooke sought my counsel again, but for a very different reason. A biopsy had revealed a suspicious-looking mole to be melanoma. As her oncologist explained, Brooke needed to go through a battery of tests to get staged—that is, to determine the severity of the disease. Then, as Brooke recalled it, she was to "get into treatment right away."

Desperate for someone to turn to, someone whom she trusted would not judge her harshly for her neediness, Brooke sat before me and cried. "I heard the words *cancer, tests, chemotherapy,* and my head began spinning," she said between sobs.

"All I could think about was my husband and my kids and my job. My brain is mush. Toni, what am I supposed to do?"

She fumbled in her purse for a crumpled piece of paper, which she handed to me. I skimmed it. All the oncologist's instructions had been written out fairly clearly. "This piece of paper . . . ," her voiced trailed off. "I can read the words, but . . . what do they mean?" And then she started to cry again—from fear and, I suspect, from the realization of just how incapacitated she had become.

I reached out and took Brooke's hand. "It's okay," I consoled her. "It's terrible news, and I know you feel hopeless and helpless right now. We can figure out what to do and how to do it together. Let me help you."

As innocuous as my words were, they seemed to cast a spell over Brooke. She allowed me to get past her defenses in a way she never had done before. I could feel her panic recede just a bit. Simply knowing that someone was there for her made a dramatic difference in her mood.

Brooke came to realize that she needed someone to lean on—and that a personal advocate could help remember what doctors were telling her and speak for her when she couldn't. If she hadn't gotten sick, she might never have gotten as close to people as she eventually did.

Teaming up with a personal advocate is a critical proactive measure in your quest to outwit cancer. It also can be an important first step in being inclusive. Throughout this book, we'll point out how the personal advocate can lend a hand with various tasks as you take control of the cancer process.

The Cancer Patient Advocate: When to Call In a Pro

Invariably, the time comes when even the cancer patient and personal advocate feel they need the input of an expert. What happens, for example, when:

- You want to get a second opinion, but you're afraid that you'll insult your doctor?

- Two doctors offer conflicting opinions, and you must choose between them?

- You want to try a complementary or alternative therapy, but you doubt that your doctor will approve?

- You need help with insurance questions?

- You've heard and read stories about exotic cures, and you're not sure what to make of them?

Usually your primary care physician serves as the point person for your medical care, coordinating the various specialists who are attending to your treatment. With cancer, however, the primary care practitioner often fades into the background as the specialists take over. This leaves a critical gap in cancer care—one that the cancer patient advocate (CPA) can bridge.

The CPA is both an informed partner and a compassionate coach, helping to manage your treatment—and your life—while encouraging you to be an active participant in the decision-making process. This person will provide information and options for all aspects of cancer care, then guide you toward informed decisions.

Different advocacy programs offer different configurations of services. Generally, the CPA can help:

- Interpret your diagnosis

- Obtain second opinions

- Assemble a medical team

- Determine an appropriate course of treatment

- Review treatment options for pain, fatigue, nausea, and other symptoms and side effects

- Search the medical literature for experimental treatments

- Select complementary and alternative medicine practitioners to provide nutrition counseling, acupuncture, massage, and other therapies as you undergo treatment

- Cut through insurance red tape

- Navigate hospital bureaucracy

- Research and arrange for rehabilitation services

- Determine posttreatment care, including necessary checkups

- Monitor for recurrence

- Make referrals for hospice and end-of-life care

Working with you and your personal advocate, the cancer patient advocate also can help manage more personal matters. Among the tasks your CPA might assist with:

- Communicating with family and friends
- Finding support services for your loved ones
- Building and managing a support network
- Dealing with anxiety and depression during treatment and recovery
- Addressing legal, financial, and employment issues
- Offering input on day-to-day personal and household matters (life management)

From Advocate to Patient

Saar became the cancer patient advocate for many of his patients, though he didn't have a name for the role at the time. Maybe it was all that rabbinic blood in him—15 generations of it. Our friends called him "a rabbi in a white coat."

As a member of the medical establishment and a cancer specialist, Saar had the expertise to share with his patients, as well as a network of peers to call upon for referrals. He knew where to find the secret buttons and levers that make the health-care system work. Mainly, though, he believed that a doctor's primary task is to be an advocate for his patients: to share knowledge, provide counsel, and offer access to the best resources around.

As Saar's reputation as an advocate grew,

he continued to shape the role. He helped patients sort through conflicting medical information by referring them for second and third opinions. He taught them to interpret research that they thought could be helpful but didn't understand. He encouraged them to investigate complementary and alternative therapies such as acupuncture and massage as adjuncts to conventional treatments. He offered direction on resolving family disagreements over medical, logistical, and lifestyle matters—and when he couldn't mediate these matters personally, he provided a referral to someone who could. He even coordinated financial assistance for indigent patients so they could get the care they needed.

Over time, Saar's collaboration with his patients revealed additional tasks with which they required guidance and support. He added these to his list of cancer patient advocate services. His patients were free to follow any of his advice—or none of it.

When Saar became sick, he had a ready-made personal advocate in me. Advocacy was my business—it's what I did as a psychologist and consultant and as an activist for political and feminist issues. Still, it took a moment of desperation for me to adapt the skills that are the cornerstone of my professional practice and apply them to what was unfolding in Saar's and my personal life.

It happened while Saar and I were meeting with Brian Durie, MD, who was affiliated with the Samuel Oschin Comprehensive Cancer Institute at Cedars-Sinai Medical Center in Los Angeles. Brian was one of a series of oncology specialists who had been recommended to us—a research and medical oncologist and a national expert in multiple myeloma.

Saar was in an advanced stage of plasma cell leukemia, the aggressive variant of multiple myeloma. Unfortunately, plasma cell leukemia is an orphan disease—one so rare that it flies beneath the radar of cancer researchers, whose limited financial resources require that they pursue only those studies that may lead to treatments for more common cancers. US doctors diagnose about 500 cases of plasma cell leukemia each year.

In Los Angeles, an expert in multiple myeloma was as close as we would get to the expertise we needed. Brian basically agreed with the other opinions we'd heard, but we intuitively liked him and wanted him to remain involved in Saar's treatment. Of course, because Brian was a national expert, his research projects took him all over the country and the world. He'd rarely be available for office visits. Though Brian was intrigued by Saar's case, Saar was pretty sick, and Brian knew we needed a medical oncologist who could be there for us on a daily basis.

I could see Saar was about ready to say, "Thanks anyway. Who do you recommend?" To my own surprise, I spoke up. "Brian, I don't want you to leave this case," I implored. "We need your expertise on plasma cell leukemia. We *need* you. How about you stay on as a consultant? How about you recommend someone to take over the daily treatment, but you remain involved for decision-making sessions at critical junctures? These could be telephone conference calls, so you can participate even while you're on the road."

Then Saar chimed in. "That sounds like a very good idea," he said. "We respect your judgment very much. It's a rather unique arrangement that Toni is suggesting, but I think it could work."

Brian had just committed to a research project that would require worldwide travel. He had to be dubious about taking on someone as sick as Saar. I could sense that he was pulling away.

"Listen," I suggested, drawing on what I knew about the politics of health care. "Cedars-Sinai delivers the best in patient-centered care in Los Angeles. You are one of the top experts in this country on this disease. You don't need to be here 100 percent. We would want to consult every couple of weeks for the first 3 months, then maybe once a month and at every crucial decision point."

Brian agreed and recommended Dan Stepan, MD, as his choice for a medical oncologist to treat Saar on a regular basis. It was a major victory. It also was a breakthrough for me. That day, I had moved beyond supporting Saar as his personal advocate to drawing on my professional skills and expertise to bring about a specific outcome. I had assumed the role of cancer patient advocate.

As we drove home, we realized that we had taken a giant step toward solidifying our medical team. With Brian as the local consulting oncologist, Dan as the treating oncologist, and Ray Alexanian, MD, of the M.D. Anderson Cancer Center in Houston willing to consult as necessary, we had assembled a team that would be able and willing to customize a

CANCER PATIENT ADVOCATE Candidate Assessment

1. What is your professional background, including your education and training?

_____

_____

2. Have you worked before as a cancer patient advocate? How often? How recently?

_____

_____

3. What is the most difficult situation you've faced as an advocate? How did you resolve it?

_____

_____

4. Have you had cancer or any other life-threatening disease? Have you lost a loved one to cancer? How can you know what I'm going through?

_____

_____

5. Are you willing to challenge or question the treatment recommendations of the doctors or hospitals I am using?

_____

_____

6. What is your fee?

_____

_____

If your primary care physician is a cancer patient advocate:

7. How will our relationship change with you as my cancer patient advocate?

_____

_____

8. What is your fee as a cancer patient advocate?

_____

_____

treatment regimen for Saar. Plus, he had a devoted personal advocate and CPA in me. Saar was in the best possible position to take control of his cancer.

PCMS Tool #1.10: Interview Your Cancer Patient Advocate

We've mentioned that choosing your personal advocate requires careful deliberation. The same is true when choosing a cancer patient advocate. Good CPAs share a number of qualities and qualifications. Interviewing candidates is the best way to find out how they measure up. This is going to be a partnership, after all.

We've put together a short list of questions (opposite) for you to use as a starting point. Feel free to add on as the conversation dictates. If you're considering having your primary care physician be your cancer patient advocate, you may want to run through these questions—especially numbers 7 and 8—to get a sense of how your doctor would fill this new role.

Declaration of Dependence

When in the course of human events that sadly lead to cancer, it becomes necessary for one patient to dissolve the walls that separate him or her from others, and to assume among the possible powers of the earth, the connected and equal station to which the Laws of Nature and of Nature's God entitle them, a decent respect to the opinions and second opinions of doctors who recommend that said patient should declare his or her dependence on those who love them.

We hold these truths to be self-evident, that all men and women are created equal, that they are endowed by their Creator with certain unalienable Rights, that among these are a healthy cancer-free Life, Liberty from pain, fatigue, and nausea, and the pursuit of happy endings. Prudence, indeed, will dictate that relationships long established should not be abandoned for light and transient ones, especially; and accordingly all experience hath shown that patient-kind are more disposed to better treatment results and to suffer less when they are aided by supportive friends and family.

I, therefore, knowing that I cannot do this alone, solemnly pledge to seek out those around me who can help me outwit cancer so that I can pursue said unalienable rights as a well person.

_____ *(Your signature here)*

_____ *(Your personal advocate's signature here)*

PCMS Tool #1.11: Sign the Declaration of Dependence

Independence is something that all of us strive for from the moment we learn to walk. Allowing ourselves to relinquish that independence—to lean on someone else for help—requires tremendous strength and self-confidence. But it's vital to your relationship with your personal advocate and your cancer patient advocate. These people depend on your trust and support, just as you depend on theirs.

To give the transfer of power an official air, you may want to read and sign the Declaration of Dependence on page 29, which loosely parallels the charter of an infant nation. Ask the person who will be your personal advocate to witness your signature.

DIVISION OF LABOR

To help track the various tasks that you will assign to yourself, your personal advocate, and your cancer patient advocate, we have included a chart like the one below at the end of every chapter. It's important to keep for yourself only those tasks that you really want to perform and have time for. As much as possible, try to delegate things to others, so you can devote your attention and energy to taking care of yourself.

TASK	WHO WILL DO IT		
	YOU	PERSONAL ADVOCATE	CPA
1. Begin collecting information from the Internet.			
2. Find a personal advocate.			
3. Interview and select a cancer patient advocate.			
4. Sign the Declaration of Dependence.			

S T E P   2

BREAK THE NEWS AND BUILD YOUR SUPPORT TEAM

When you found out that you have cancer, your first instinct probably was to be alone—to hide out somewhere and nurse your wounds. But you can't do that for long. Instead, you need to figure out how to stay a step ahead of your diagnosis. Your goals are simple but gigantic: Find a cure for your cancer, and keep going until you do. That means identifying your needs, organizing your time, and finding people to assist you.

It's a lot to expect of yourself, especially at such a stressful time. When you most feel like running away from everything, stop, take a breath, and congratulate yourself on the progress you're making. Then move on. There are benefits to immersing yourself in the battle rather than retreating from it. As the Alcoholics Anonymous slogan says, "When I got busy, I got better."

The caveat, of course, is to get busy in a meaningful way. Now is not the time to overextend yourself or to invest your time and energy in unproductive tasks. By following the steps of the Personal Cancer Management System (PCMS), you'll be able to home in on the essentials and let go of the rest.

You may encounter some PCMS tools that don't seem especially practical or productive. Please try them anyway. Often the thing that seems the least promising is the one that produces the best results. Solutions to problems come from unlikely places. Plan to be surprised by what you can do to take control of your illness—and how the very act of planning can transform your world.

In this step, your first task is to share your news. You may agonize about how to go about it; just do whatever seems right. In most cases, you will tell your spouse or partner first, then your children and best friends, your siblings and parents, and the rest of your immediate family. Acquaintances will come next, then finally your co-workers. Once the word is out, you can go about the business of assembling your support team.

An old European parable tells of a penniless but resourceful man who is trying to get something to eat. He finds a cauldron, fills it with water, and sets it over a fire. To passersby, he says he's making soup. He doesn't mention that his own contribution to the ingredients is a stone he's put in the water; a stone is all he has.

The first person who stops is a man with a fond recollection of cabbage soup. He fetches a cabbage. Another remembers soup with salt beef, and he happens to have a bit of beef. A woman who has just pulled a few carrots throws them in the pot. Others bring onions, salt and pepper, garlic, potatoes,

beets, barley—whatever they have on hand.

So the man who started with little more than an idea and a cauldron ends up with a hearty, nourishing soup. His tale illustrates the value of collective action—how we can achieve so much more by combining resources and becoming a community.

Sometimes a serious illness such as cancer can unite people as nothing else can. It can elicit from others a generosity that they did not know they possessed. At some point in the cancer process, you will bring out the best in someone by asking for that person's help and support. Remember this as you go about the task of telling others and inviting them to be part of your support team.

BREAK THE NEWS

It's hard enough when you find out that you have cancer. Now you must tell those whom you hold dearest and risk breaking their hearts in the process.

More than likely, the news will get out to some people who you'd prefer didn't know about it. You also may find that once your personal misfortune becomes public knowledge, you attract people with their own stories of misfortune, people who feel like victims and who want to establish common cause. If they depress or distract you, feel free to avoid them. You need to focus on yourself right now.

Cancer comes into your life much as a new in-law comes into a family, shaking up every relationship. Even your family and friends may provoke stress. "Who needs this?" you ask, as you take steps to isolate yourself from them. You make elaborate excuses to avoid calling them. You believe that you're keeping your illness a secret because you want to protect them or because you don't want to burden them with your problem. You decide that you'll open up to them when you have good news or when the timing is better. But once you knock down that wall of resistance, the love and support you get back will more than compensate for the difficulty of breaking the news for the first time.

Why is talking about cancer so hard to do? A key reason is that we learn from an early age to value rugged individualism. None of us likes to admit to needing help from others. We strive to be independent. In psychology, the developmental stage known as individuation is about separating our identities from our parents'. It's a sign of growth and maturity.

The United States achieved maturity by declaring its independence from England. Culturally we do the same. We idolize and idealize "self-made men"—loners like James Dean, Clint Eastwood, and other macho male movie stars. We have spent a generation redefining femininity to encourage women to also be independent, adding careers and breadwinning to traditional familial roles.

Self-sufficiency works for some things some of the time. In our experience, it probably won't help get you through a serious health crisis. A true sign of personal strength is to find a new way to operate, one that leaves the "rugged" out of rugged individualism and views reliance on others as a virtue. As 17th-century English poet and preacher

John Donne wrote, "No man is an island, entire of itself; every man is a piece of the continent, a part of the main."

Those who allow themselves the flexibility to be dependent often can do so only when they feel independence in other areas of their lives. Here's a task for you: Make the other aspects of your life so strong, so secure that you can reach out to others without feeling weak. You'll recognize your reluctance to ask for help as a resistor and overcome that block.

And if you didn't sign the Declaration of Dependence at the end of Step 1 (page 29), go back and do so now. The rest of the PCMS will be much easier.

How to Tell People

Even for naturally inclusive extroverts, finding the right words to disclose a cancer diagnosis can be a challenge. It may seem awkward at first, so take a little time to think through what you're going to say. Try not to obsess about it, though. It will get easier as you go along.

When Saar and I decided to tell others about his cancer, we figured that we might as well tackle the toughest audience first. So we arranged a meeting with his daughter, Laura; her husband, Randy; and my son, Mitch, all of whom live near us. (Saar's other daughter, Ellen, lives in New York. He thought that a one-on-one conversation might work better for her.)

There is no easy way to tell your children that you have a life-threatening illness. Your kids look to you as their pillars of strength,

Alan had sought out my consulting organization, the Leadership Equation Institute, when he needed help with succession planning as his company went through the transition from family business to corporate entity. All went smoothly, and at age 50, he was well positioned for the future. Though he consulted me from time to time, I assumed our important work was done.

Then I got a message from him. When he came into my office, we spent some time catching up. From the sound of things, his company was doing fine. He was especially pleased with Don, the man who had come onboard as president and who would succeed him as CEO.

"So what was the concern I heard in your voice?" I finally asked. "Is there the threat of a takeover, some kind of scandal?"

"Toni, it's worse," Alan said, leaning forward as though he feared the room might be bugged. "I have lung cancer, and it doesn't look good. I've told my wife and kids—that was no picnic—but now how do I tell the folks at work?" He explained the details of his illness and the emotional and medical support that he and his family had already put in place. His family was as prepared as it could be. His consternation really was about his colleagues.

At that point, Alan pulled out an organizational chart that showed his leadership group by their functional positions and by his relationship to them. His concern was how to tell Don, because Alan needed him to remain committed to the company and its future.

I reminded Alan of RECE (recognize, empathize, collaborate, empower), an exercise he had learned through the Leader-

and though they may see you in times of weakness and vulnerability, they believe you will always be there for them—sometimes quite literally. Even grown children have a sense that their parents are immortal. And we parents want to live up to that expectation.

Like all families, ours had issues. The question was, could we set aside the anger, hurt, and mistrust from the past to deal with the crisis at hand?

For Laura and Randy, this would mean not giving in to a sense of misfortune. Randy's father, Mike, had been diagnosed with inoperable pancreatic cancer a few months earlier. They had moved up their wedding to make sure Mike could be there. Now it appeared that on their first anniversary, both of their fathers might be gone. Their children might not have grandfathers.

As for Mitch, he needed to come to terms with years of strained emotions that we hoped he could let go. His father and I had divorced when he was a teenager. Then Saar came into my life. Mitch loved Saar's reliability but struggled with his rough edge.

We invited the kids to come over on a

ship Equation program. Together, we crafted another version of it that Alan could use in his current situation.

After some rehearsing, Alan set up a meeting with Don. Using RECE, he told his colleague about his cancer. Expecting things to go smoothly, Alan was shocked when Don said, "I'm sorry you're sick, but you told me I'd move up in 3 to 5 years. It's only 18 months. I'm just not ready."

Sticking with his RECE script, Alan empathized with Don and encouraged him to open up about his concerns. Even more than his lack of experience, Don was worried about a potential conflict between himself and an executive vice president who had her eye on the CEO spot. He was nervous about the entire succession process.

Alan thought he'd be able to focus on his treatment without worrying about his com-pany. Now his corporate "dream team" was falling apart. He came back to me, and we talked further. He agreed that to allay Don's (and his own) concerns, he would need to get very specific—affirming Don's strengths while empathizing with his concerns about competition and his fear about not being ready. Don was seeking reassurance that his promotion would not be perceived as opportunistic and that he would not be expected to be perfect right out of the gate.

The two agreed to set up weekly succession meetings to plan all contingencies, as well as to appoint a seasoned advisory board and enlist executive coaching as a backup. An exit strategy that established Don as the CEO was already in place. Now they had time to reinforce it. Their collaboration served as a model for the company's new way of doing business.

Wednesday night. They arrived on guard; a midweek, mandatory-attendance family dinner tends to send up a red flag. We gathered in the library, a snug room at the center of our home.

"I have something important to tell you," Saar started tentatively, sitting in his favorite recliner, his command post.

"Like we didn't know that," Laura broke in. "You invite us to dinner on a weekday night, and you sound so mysterious." Everyone laughed. Laughter is good.

Saar explained that he had not been up to snuff of late, then proceeded with a lengthy explanation that sounded like a lot of medical mumbo-jumbo. He went into great detail about symptoms and medical tests, not giving anyone a chance to interrupt.

"What are you *saying*, Dad?" Laura finally interjected.

"I may have plasma cell leukemia," he replied. "It's a type of cancer."

Mitch nodded, as though he was trying to find some sort of hopeful signal. Randy grimaced. This was déjà vu for him. Laura, who thinks like her father, started firing off questions. "So what did the doctors say? What are you going to do next? What is the chance of survival? What sort of treatment—chemotherapy or radiation therapy? What are the side effects? Are you getting a second opinion? From whom? When? Where?"

Saar would put up a good fight, he assured them, but he needed their help. Then he broke down and cried. One by one, the kids hugged him or held his hand or stroked his head, as though their touch would make the nightmare go away. It was like a scene from an old war movie, where the person in command announces he's going to battle and asks who will join him, knowing he needs everyone.

PCMS Tool #2.1: Practice Your Conversation

Admittedly, Saar and I had stumbled through that first telling relatively unprepared, though it turned out okay in the end. Still, some advance planning couldn't hurt. Think about it: When we're teenagers, we can't ask for a date without practicing what we'll say. As we get older, we do "dry runs" of job interviews, marriage proposals, and important conversations with our kids. Why stop now?

Beyond rehearsing, the following strategies can help make breaking the news a little bit easier.

• Contact those most important and closest to you first. If you can, arrange to meet in person. Otherwise, leave a phone message asking for a time when the two of you can talk. Say simply, "I have something important to share

with you. Let me know when you're free." If phone calls or face-to-face meetings can't be arranged, send an e-mail instead.

• If you are able to get together in person, pick a time and place where neither of you will be interrupted by phones, faxes, e-mails, children, spouses, or anything else. Sit in the park, a coffee shop, or even your car. Make sure you allow enough time; your conversation may take longer than you expect.

• Avoid starting the conversation by blurting out, "I have cancer." Try not to get caught up in small talk, either; you'll digress and never get back to the subject. Instead, you might want to ease into the news of your diagnosis by presenting events chronologically, in the order leading up to your diagnosis. For example: "I haven't been feeling too well lately, so I went to see my doctor. The test results showed some irregularities in my blood work. So my doctor referred me to a specialist, who confirmed that something may be wrong. I had another test, which found a tumor. It looks malignant. I may have cancer, but I will be going for more tests next week. Meanwhile, we're exploring all the options, and we want to get a second opinion."

Often people prefer to deal with cancer as a medical diagnosis and not as a sign from God or a death sentence from the medical establishment.

Drawing on our experience in talking to our children, a little medical detail can go a very long way.

- Be prepared to elaborate with whatever facts you have collected and feel comfortable sharing: the type of cancer, your doctors, the treatment options, your immediate plan of action.

- Don't sugarcoat the prognosis, but don't be overly pessimistic, either. Cautiously hopeful is a wonderful approach. It's also accurate.

- Be honest and open. People will respond in kind.

- Forgive ignorance. Despite the prevalence of cancer, many people still harbor misconceptions about it. They may think, for example, that it's contagious. Enlighten them without being condescending.

- End with a request. You might say, "I may ask for your help from time to time. Someone will need to take me for treatments, pick up groceries, help out with the kids, that sort of thing. Mostly, I just need you to be here for me. And if you can take on a task, like driving me to the doctor's office or picking up the kids a couple of times a week, that would be terrific."

After you've run through this conversation once or twice, throw away the script. When great actors describe their work, they rarely talk about diction and emotion and intellect. They talk about listening to the other actor and responding truthfully. Your success with a script probably depends less on what you're saying than on what you're able to hear.

- When talking with someone, set aside whatever else you may be doing. Focus on the person and the messages, verbal and nonverbal, that he or she is sending.

- Make and maintain eye contact, but don't stare. Concentrating on the person's eye color may help.

- Give the person a chance to respond. Ask questions instead of making statements. Questions soften the conversation by engaging the other person. They initiate dialogue and facilitate a two-way exchange. Remember, you will want this person's support.

- Don't jump in at the first break in the conversation. It sounds as if you're not listening—as if you're standing at the starting line waiting for the gun to go off, so you can speak again.

- Don't smile constantly. It may be meant to look friendly, but often it's interpreted as spacing out or not taking the other person seriously.

By the way, you may be surprised at how people respond to the news of your illness. They may seem to be reacting more strongly than you are. Despite their best intentions, some family members or friends will have trouble staying close to you when you need them most.

When Saar became ill, one of his patients, Regina Manfridi, wrote to him, describing how she had struggled to come to terms with his diagnosis. "I remember when I had cancer, people stayed away from me as if I were contagious," she recalled. "Others tried to reduce [my illness] to the value of a cold or tried to erase it from my mind. Others couldn't find the right words and so said nothing. I know what they were feeling. Words seem so inadequate."

In our work as cancer patient advocates, we've seen and heard about all sorts of unexpected reactions from people who learn that a loved one has cancer. Here's how to handle these situations.

- Anticipate questions to which you may or may not have answers. Some people, like Laura, may ask questions as an intellectual buffer to the fear and sadness they feel. Provide as much information as you can. If you don't know all the answers, don't sweat it. You're just learning yourself. Moreover, some things about cancer baffle even the top experts. If someone has a good question, write it down and ask your doctor.

- Don't protect anyone. Some family members and friends may seem to need your support more than you need theirs. For them, hearing the word *cancer* may trigger fears of loss and mortality. Don't use the weakness of those who are close to you as an excuse not to tell them. If they fall apart, they fall apart. Just be careful not to resent them if they do. Once they see your strength in telling them, they'll rise to the occasion. Notice how children react in a crisis; they won't cry if the adults

around them stay calm. We're all like that, no matter how old we are.

- Be ready for tears. And hugs. And more of the same. Remember that emotions are natural and expressing them is healthy. They are signs not of weakness but of strength. This is no time to expect those you tell, or even yourself, to put up a brave front or play hero. You'll have plenty of time for that later on. For you and for those closest to you, breaking down may be the healthiest response. Saying "Don't cry" has never stopped anyone from crying. What's more, it denies the person the right to experience an honest emotion.

- Accept rejection. If people turn down your request for assistance, don't take it personally. They probably are fleeing from their own fear. Don't turn your back on them. They may think you're withdrawing from them. Once they have a chance to mull over your news, they may change their minds and offer help.

- Don't be offended. If you have waited a couple of weeks before telling a family member or friend, that person may respond indignantly, "How long have you known this?" The implication is, "I'm hurt and insulted that you didn't tell me sooner. I thought we were closer than that." Finding fault with some detail is what people do when they can't comprehend the whole situation. Keep them up-to-date, but give them space to work through their feelings. They will absorb your news in stages, at their own pace. Just remember to leave the door open to them; they may be helpful later on.

- Be prepared to make assignments. Many people will offer help. It's not a bad idea to think about what you'll be needing and even who might best handle each particular task. We'll discuss this in more detail later in the chapter.

Guy Talk

Disclosing a serious illness such as cancer may come a bit easier to women than to men. From a young age, women seek empathy and connection in their relationships. Men are looking for buddies—someone to shoot a round of golf with but not necessarily confide in. They're reluctant to engage in deeply personal conversations, even with other men whom they've known for a long time. It's an unfortunate by-product of their learned tendency to withhold their emotions.

Saar grew up envying the closeness between his sister and her friends. Early on, he decided that he would form deeper bonds in his friendships. He wrote:

Most boys grow up with a couple of close friends, plus a larger group or club for hanging out. As we get older, our friendships give way to lots of superficial acquaintances. I was lucky to be close to six great guys. If I would have gone out of town for my treatments, any and all of them would have offered to take off a week at a time to be there with me. When I became dis-

abled, they would have given me money if I had needed it, which fortunately I didn't.

Lee and Lenny probably were the most empathetic of the group—Lee because he had been through many bouts of ulcerative colitis (one of them life-threatening), and Lenny because he'd had coronary angioplasty. Life-threatening events really do change people—at least, if people allow them to, as in the case of Lee and Lenny.

Not all of Saar's friends reacted in the same way. In fact, Saar found telling one friend—perhaps his closest—to be particularly difficult. Although Saar and Irwin shared much in common, they were opposites in one important way. Irwin is an introvert; he never expresses his emotions. Saar lets it all hang out.

Because Irwin is a physician, Saar told him the diagnosis point-blank, doctor to doctor. Irwin didn't react at all, at least visibly. He was very quiet at first. Then both men shifted into the medical mind-set, objectively analyzing the diagnosis and the options.

Saar's one request of Irwin was to not tell his wife, Ellen. She and I are very close. Both Saar and I thought she should hear the news from me.

After their conversation, Saar didn't hear from Irwin for several days. So he called his friend. "Hey, how are you?" Saar asked. "I hope you're not going to disappear on me now that I really need you."

"No," was all Irwin could get out before he choked up.

The news of Saar's cancer had affected Irwin so deeply that he seemed to have gone into a minor state of shock. He withdrew not just from Saar but from his wife, his work, his world. He said he couldn't concentrate; he tried to read, but his mind was somewhere else, going in circles.

"Do you mind if I tell Ellen?" Irwin finally asked. He needed an outlet, someone to talk to.

"Sure," Saar replied, "if you think you might be able to deal with it better."

The next afternoon, Irwin and Ellen came to our house. They wanted nothing more than to announce their unequivocal support. They were in this together, with us.

"Thank God," Saar said afterward. "Now that he's accepted some of his own pain and suffering, he can be there for me."

Everyone has his or her own tolerances and limits, learning style, and coping strategy. Try not to let this bother you. In the end, all you want is for those closest to you to be there for you.

Disclosure in the Workplace

Opening up to your colleagues about your cancer diagnosis is a more sensitive matter. You may worry that you're no longer a contributing member of the workforce, that you are seen as damaged goods. You may fear, perhaps rightly so, that your news will become a topic of gossip rather than a conduit for strengthening workplace bonds.

Some people will resent being called upon to pick up some of your workload. Others may start vying for your position well before you are ready to quit. Clients, worried that you won't be able to follow through on commitments, may talk about taking their business elsewhere. If you're in a management or executive position, you may worry that the delicate chain of command you've established to protect your own power base will collapse in your absence.

Relationships with co-workers are quite different from those with family and friends. Since you spend most of your waking hours with these people, they may seem like extended family. But often the workplace is a highly politicized, Machiavellian environment. Until now, you may have chosen to keep your personal life to yourself. You never wanted to show your vulnerability when the guy in the cubicle next to yours or a fellow member of the management team could be after your position. Now things have changed. You will need to build on all the alliances you have established.

Make sure that the people closest to you hear the news directly from you—or, if that isn't possible, from someone who can speak on your behalf. With bad news, especially, people need to hear it from the right source. As for who should know first, it's customary to start at the top, with your boss. This is just smart office politics. You wouldn't want the person who holds the purse strings to find out secondhand.

Once you've talked with your boss, you can tell your most trusted colleagues, then move on from there. The following pointers should help the process go smoothly.

- As you share the news with your colleagues, ask that they keep it to themselves until you've had a chance to speak with everyone directly.

- If you deal with clients and customers outside the office, decide ahead of time just how much you want them to know.

- Try to tell people over as short a period of time as possible. The rumor mill grinds very quickly, as you probably know.

- Make arrangements to meet your colleagues outside the office—perhaps after work at a local café. Don't expect them to drop what they're doing, listen to what you have to say, and then pick up where they left off.

- If you can't meet after work, plan your conversations for as close to the end of the day as possible. Your news will be emotionally exhausting. That way your colleagues—and you—can go home and recover.

PCMS Tool #2.2: Use RECE to Communicate Effectively

The acronym RECE stands for *r*ecognize, *e*mpathize, *c*ollaborate, *e*mpower. It's a strategy for interacting with people so that your message gets across to them and their response comes through clearly to you. Most important, it teaches you to use empathy to create an effective communication loop whenever one is necessary. Empathy, research teaches us, is the most powerful communication technique we have.

On page 42, we've included a sample for you, so you can see how RECE works in practice. Make as many copies of the blank worksheet on page 43 as you wish, so you can

use it when you need to prepare for potentially awkward or difficult conversations.

Telling Others Helps You

Since you're the patient, it may seem odd that we're spending so much time on those around you—their emotions, their reactions, their interactions with you. That's less paradoxical than it seems. Being human, you are a social animal. You'll be asking those closest to you for help. They'll play a major role in your care.

Therefore, everything you do to help those around you weather this crisis is good for you, too. A dark secret is a heavy burden. Trying to disguise the fact that you're afraid or that you feel sick will wear on you and slow your recovery. So even if a few conversations don't go as well as you hoped, continue to tell those who need to know about your diagnosis. It's to your advantage in the long run.

BUILD YOUR SUPPORT TEAM

Remember that as you break the news of your illness, you are enlisting those around you to join your support team. They're vital to helping you through what lies ahead. In the course of your conversations, you may discover that some whom you thought you could count on can't or won't be there for you, while others will demonstrate insights, ideas, and reserves of character that you didn't expect.

We've created a series of tools to help you organize your support team. Let's walk through each one in turn.

41

(continued on page 45)

USE RECE TO COMMUNICATE EFFECTIVELY

Telling Your Boss

RECOGNIZE

FOCUS ON THE OTHER PERSON'S NEEDS AND MESSAGES RATHER THAN TRYING TO BE HEARD. ASK QUESTIONS RATHER THAN OFFERING OPINIONS.

Tom, you've always said that you want me to come to you first and fast with important issues, so you aren't caught off guard. I always try to remember that. Now I need to tell you something. I recently found out that I have cancer. I wanted you to know before anyone else here. I'd love to get your input on how best to break the news to the rest of the team.

EMPATHIZE AND ENGAGE

LISTEN MORE, TALK LESS. USE INTERACTIONS TO BUILD BRIDGES. MAKE A HUMAN CONNECTION BY EXTENDING YOURSELF TO SHOW INTEREST IN THE OTHER PERSON.

I know you need to put the company first, and I agree.

COLLABORATE

BE SPECIFIC. EMPHASIZE THE POSITIVE AND USE THAT AS LEVERAGE FOR COMING TO RESOLUTION.

I've laid out a contingency plan to ensure that the work gets done if and when I'm not here. It needs tightening, especially in the sales area. I'd appreciate your feedback. You're great at strategizing when problems like this arise.

EMPOWER

RECOGNIZE THE OTHER PERSON'S IDEAS, SKILLS, AND ABILITY TO MOVE FORWARD.

You're the only one who can give the green light to this plan. Please take a look at it, and let me know if it works for you and the company.

USE RECE TO COMMUNICATE EFFECTIVELY

_____

RECOGNIZE

FOCUS ON THE OTHER PERSON'S NEEDS AND MESSAGES RATHER THAN TRYING TO BE HEARD. ASK QUESTIONS RATHER THAN OFFERING OPINIONS.

_____
_____
_____

EMPATHIZE AND ENGAGE

LISTEN MORE, TALK LESS. USE INTERACTIONS TO BUILD BRIDGES. MAKE A HUMAN CONNECTION BY EXTENDING YOURSELF TO SHOW INTEREST IN THE OTHER PERSON.

_____
_____
_____

COLLABORATE

BE SPECIFIC. EMPHASIZE THE POSITIVE AND USE THAT AS LEVERAGE FOR COMING TO RESOLUTION.

_____
_____
_____

EMPOWER

RECOGNIZE THE OTHER PERSON'S IDEAS, SKILLS, AND ABILITY TO MOVE FORWARD.

_____
_____
_____

Sharon and Norman's Tag Team

Sharon was a long-term patient of Saar's. Early on, he served as her cancer patient advocate, helping her to tell her husband, Norman, that she had breast cancer. "I want to tell him, but I don't think I can tell him alone," she explained. "It will break his heart . . . and mine. Norman expects us to be the perfect couple."

Saar invited the couple to his office, where he proceeded to break the news to Norman. Saar was patient, logical, and compassionate. He reviewed the options for further testing and treatment as well as the various decisions Sharon and Norman would need to make.

Of course, Norman was devastated. But hearing it in the protected environment of Saar's office and hearing it from a doctor who objectively laid out the entire situation lessened the blow. Norman surprised Sharon by enlisting. "We're in this together, honey, whatever happens," he said.

Afterward, Sharon told Saar, "I feel dumb for assuming that Norman would be mad at me for ruining our 'perfect' reputation and that he'd love me less." When Norman showed that he could handle the problem, Sharon became sure she could handle it, too. "We'll beat this thing, Doc," she said.

Then came Norman's turn. Several years after Sharon's diagnosis, a routine physical revealed Norman's high PSA count. Further tests confirmed that he had prostate cancer. He came to Saar. "How am I going to tell Sharon?" he confided, forgetting or maybe never knowing that she had sat in the same chair and asked a similar question.

Saar knew from his experience and conversations with Sharon that she could handle the news bravely. Norman was the worrier. He resisted acknowledging imperfection in his life. He had stood by Sharon through her cancer, but he didn't deal with his own illness all that well. He perceived it as a flaw, a weakness.

Saar thought that the best strategy for helping Norman would be to show him how he was getting in his own way. Norman's assignment was to work through a series of exercises to help recognize and overcome patterns of resistance to being inclusive. In a way, Saar was challenging Norman to aim for excellence by using the exercises to expose and deal with his illness.

Norman's resistance weakened further when Sharon took on the role of caregiver and personal advocate in the same way that Norman had done for her. As a consequence, Norman learned a great deal about himself. He told Saar that he needed to practice including other people "if I'm going to get good at it."

He did get good at it. Today, both Norman and Sharon are cancer survivors. And they're still married.

PCMS Tool #2.3: Create Your Circle of Supporters

Your support team consists of the people with whom you will interact on a daily basis. It might be three or four people or a dozen. At the center, of course, are you and your personal advocate. As we discussed in Step 1 (page 19), your personal advocate is someone close to you—a spouse, a sibling, an adult child, or a best friend—who will be there for you, fighting alongside you whenever you need another set of eyes or ears, another voice, another presence.

Among the primary functions of your support team is assisting with essential everyday tasks. In the beginning, this may mean making phone calls for you or taking walks with you. Over time, your support team may take on other responsibilities such as preparing your meals, watching your children, feeding and walking your pets, and escorting you to and from doctor's appointments.

You'll be spending a lot of time with the members of your support team, so consider not only how well someone can perform specific tasks but also how comfortable you feel with that person. Don't include Barbara, the great chauffeur, if she gets on your nerves. You really won't be able to tolerate her behavior while you're under so much stress.

Looking at the diagram on page 46, think about whom you would include and where they fit in. Jot down names as appropriate. Each circle represents a different group and role. You may have whole categories of potential supporters we haven't mentioned—members of your church, PTA, or book club, or friends with whom you bowl or travel.

Immediate family: This category includes your spouse or partner, children, parents, siblings, and all other close relatives. They can be your pillars of support, and they'll want to know how they can help. But they'll need your guidance.

Close friends: They are your emotional safety net. You may find yourself asking them just to be there for you, for walks or late-night phone calls or an occasional night out. They're also your bench, as they say in basketball—the backup squad that steps in when things get tough.

Extended family: This group draws from your wider circle of friends and acquaintances. They are cousins, neighbors, or old classmates from across the country. When they ask if they can do anything, you can say, "Just check in when you can, and keep me in your prayers."

Co-workers: They can be close friends or purely professional associates. What they are able to provide for you will vary. You may need someone to fill in for you while you're at a doctor's appointment or to research your company's health benefits and medical leave policy. Or perhaps you just want another person you can turn to for support.

Cancer patient advocate: As explained in Step 1, a cancer patient advocate (CPA) can provide invaluable support through every step of your cancer treatment and care, from choosing doctors and getting second opinions to gathering information on clinical trials. Your primary care physician may have the training to take on this role. If not, and if you want a CPA on your support team, you'll need to broaden your search.

Others: This group includes anyone who doesn't fit into one of the above categories—pharmacists, wig makers, people you know from your gym or met in your doctor's waiting room. They may turn out to be some of your most helpful resources.

PCMS Tool #2.4: Collect Contact Information

Now that you've made a chart of your supporters, your next task is to put the information into a more user-friendly format. A list is

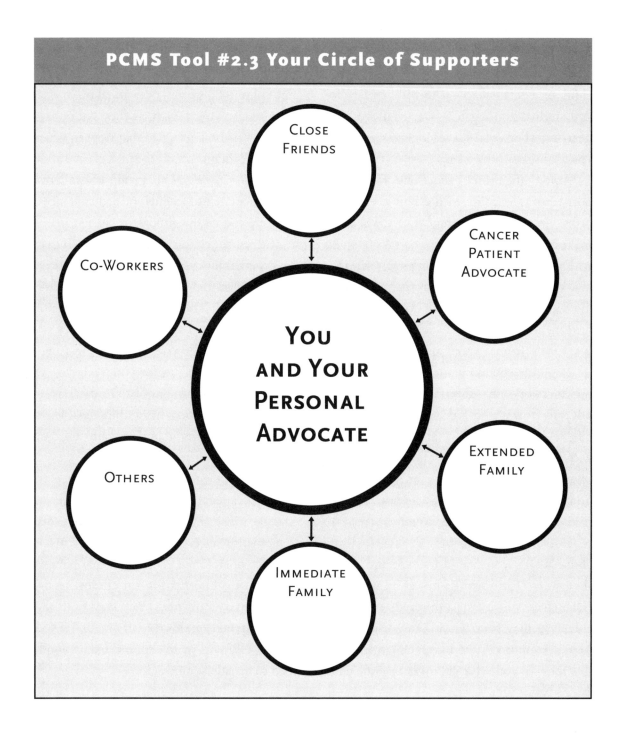

PCMS Tool #2.3 Your Circle of Supporters

CLOSE FRIENDS

CANCER PATIENT ADVOCATE

CO-WORKERS

YOU AND YOUR PERSONAL ADVOCATE

EXTENDED FAMILY

OTHERS

IMMEDIATE FAMILY

a good tool for this purpose—compact but expandable.

Everyone makes lists differently. We've included a very basic form on page 48, which you can photocopy. You might prefer to store this information in a daily planner, on your laptop, or in a Palm Pilot. Or you might take a more low-tech route—a tablet or even the back of an envelope.

What's most important is that you keep the names and contact information for every member of your support team in one place. You might want to group them in broad categories, such as:

- Those to call in case of emergency
- Those who provide specific services, such as child care
- Those to contact for comfort and advice

Be sure to update contact information as it changes. And make lots of copies, so you can place a list wherever you might need to access one—at home, at work, and in your purse or briefcase.

PCMS Tool #2.5: Assign Tasks

As you were filling in the chart of your supporters, you probably had some ideas about who could do what for you. Now is a good time to compile a list of those tasks and to make tentative assignments (page 49). They may change once you gather your support team for a meeting (which we'll discuss next). For the time being, this list will provide a helpful visual of just what needs to be done.

Right now, you may be preoccupied with

what lies ahead, in terms of your cancer diagnosis. The fact is, the rest of your life will be as hectic and demanding as ever. You will need to juggle other ongoing obligations—to your family, to your employer, to your community—with your cancer treatment, which will become close to a full-time job.

PCMS Tool #2.6: Create a Buddy System

With your lists of supporters and assignments in hand, you're ready to officially appoint your support team. Here's what to do.

1. Using your lists as guides, select a co-ordinator. It should be someone who is responsible and organized and who has the time, energy, and interest to serve as your point person. Call and find out if this person would be willing to assume the role of coordinator. Explain that the job would entail contacting the rest of your supporters to find out if they're willing to become your "buddies," and then creating and implementing an assignment schedule.

2. Once you've appointed a coordinator, ask this person to call or e-mail each of your prospective buddies. Your coordinator can explain that the two of you are in the process of assembling a support team, then ask the following questions.

   - How much time do you have available for this?
   - Are you capable of managing household tasks from cleaning to cooking?

(continued on page 50)

COLLECT CONTACT INFORMATION

My Supporters

Name	Contact Information (phone number, fax number, e-mail address, street address)
1.	
2.	
3.	
4.	
5.	
6.	
7.	
8.	
9.	
10.	
11.	
12.	

ASSIGN TASKS

Support Team Assignments

Jobs and Responsibilities	Name	Availability
Sample: Drive to doctor's appointment		
Sample: Pick up kids at school		
Sample: Prepare meals		

- Will you do childcare if needed?

- Can you do Internet research?

- Would you attend doctors' appointments and feel comfortable asking questions and taking notes?

- Would you provide care during treatment and recovery?

- How comfortable are you with managing a sick person's physical needs?

- Are you good at completing insurance forms, checking on payments, making follow-up calls, and writing letters about claims?

- Would you write thank-you notes and return calls to well-wishers?

3. Ask your coordinator to arrange a meeting with all of your prospective buddies. Though an in-person meeting is best, you can gather by phone or online, if that's more convenient for everyone.

4. Prior to the meeting, schedule an appointment with your coordinator so the two of you can review your lists of supporters and tasks. Send copies of these documents to all of your prospective buddies as well.

5. Start the meeting by thanking everyone for coming. Tell them that because they are so important to you, you have brought them together to help you in your fight against cancer. Introduce your coordinator, who can then explain his or her role, as well as the support team assignments. Your assignment list will illustrate how this group effort will be critical during your treatment and care.

6. Leave the room (virtually or actually) and let your coordinator run the next segment of the meeting, which is reviewing the tasks and the people chosen to perform them. At this time, the coordinator can ask if each person is able to take on the assigned tasks; if not, then substitute volunteers can be requested. The coordinator can work through the entire list in this manner, jotting down notes and checking the list to make sure that every task is taken care of.

7. When you rejoin the group, thank everyone for attending the meeting. Tell them that they will receive an updated schedule and contact list, reflecting the changes from the meeting, and that the coordinator will keep in touch with them by phone, fax, or e-mail. You might consider presenting a thank-you token to each person, such as a laminated button or pen with your name on it—e.g., "Sally's Supporters."

For more information on creating a buddy system, visit www.drhaber.com, the Web site of Sandra Haber, PhD. She is a clinical psychologist and trained cancer patient advocate practicing in New York City. She is also on the faculty of the Porrath Foundation for Cancer Patient Advocacy training program.

Building Support Is a Continuous Process

Putting your support team together is important; keeping it together is even more so. You need to develop and nurture those relationships that will sustain you in the weeks and months ahead. Saar liked to quote a line attributed to the great statesman Pericles in *The History of the Peloponnesian War:* "We secure our friends not by accepting favors but by doing them."

This doesn't mean that people will turn their backs on you if you can't keep giving. In the best relationships, a gift given is indistinguishable from a gift received. Think of the best present you ever gave to someone you really care about. Who derived the most pleasure from it? You may be giving enough by asking for help; it creates an opportunity for a loved one to give in return.

One way to show appreciation to those on your support team is to keep them posted on your progress. They're donating their time and energy to your cause; they are hoping that their effort is of benefit. Even if you don't have good news, a "progress report" will be welcome. People need reassurance that you want them in your life.

Of course, keeping in touch is difficult under the best of circumstances. It can seem impossible now, as you want to preserve your strength and manage your stress. In this context, nurturing your support team may seem like one more tiring responsibility. When you consider the return in love, kindness, and positive energy, it is certainly worth the investment.

PCMS Tool #2.7: Write a "Dear Everybody" Letter

Saar and I came up with the idea of a "Dear Everybody" letter as a solution to a dilemma.

We understood that people wanted to stay abreast of Saar's progress. And we wanted to share the news—the results of doctors' visits, tests, and all the rest. We would have liked to personally call or write each person who helped us, with a note asking how things were going in their lives. But we were so overwhelmed by the ongoing challenges of Saar's illness that sometimes all we could do was catch up with each other at the end of the day. So we decided to write one letter, photocopy it, and send it to everyone who had asked us to stay in touch. Today, you could do this by e-mail.

The "Dear Everybody" is like one of those letters that some families send out at the holidays, catching up with other family members and friends on the year's accomplishments ("Timmy took his first steps," "Jessica got into Princeton," "Don's tomatoes won first prize in the county fair"). Only our letter wasn't about blue ribbons and college acceptances.

You don't need to be Shakespeare to draft a good letter to your family and friends. Simply write with honesty, love, and gratitude. As we learned, what you say doesn't matter all that much anyway. People just want to feel your presence.

The letters, which you can send out from time to time throughout your cancer treatment, allow you to thank everyone at once. They save dozens of phone calls. They can be more personal, too. Writing allows you to express deep feelings that may not come out as comfortably or eloquently over the phone or in person. People will appreciate your taking the time to put your updates in a form that they can keep and reread as they wish.

The content of your letter can be anything you want. These tips might help simplify the task.

- Share the responsibility with someone else. Some people love to write; others loathe it. If you can't find a volunteer, you might try recording your thoughts on a tape player and transcribing the tape. Then all your letter needs is some editing and polishing.

- Give an update on your condition, but not necessarily in detailed clinical terminology. Explain what has happened so far and what will happen next. Don't leave things hanging or try to create suspense; your phone will be ringing off the hook.

- Report on things other than your illness to show that cancer isn't consuming your entire life. Talk about your pets, your garden, or your golf score.

- Be honest about your feelings, hopes, and fears. It's not necessary to be a Pollyanna or to put on a good face. People know you, and they know cancer is no day at the beach.

- Close your letter with more thanks to your family and friends for their continued help and support through these challenging times. Let them know that they should keep the good wishes coming and that you'll holler if you need more.

Besides letters, you have other ways of maintaining the connection to your support team. For example:

A phone tree: Along with a "Dear Everybody" letter, a phone tree can keep the members of your support team communicating with each other. Ask your team coordinator to divvy the names of your supporters among several people. Then they can call everyone on their respective phone lists with updates on your treatment and other news.

E-mail: Create a special group mailing list. You can send your "Dear Everybody" letter as an attachment.

A Web site: Choose and register an Internet domain name, then recruit someone to design and manage the site for you. You can post recent photos, inspirational quotes, and links to other Web sites with information ranging from the types of treatment you're getting to the books you're reading, such as this one!

PCMS Tool #2.8: Change Your Phone Message

You'll be getting countless calls from well-wishers as you progress from cancer diagnosis through treatment. But sometimes, after spending hours trying to obtain test results or resolve an insurance claim, chatting on the phone is the last thing you want to do—even when it's with the family members and friends who are your lifeline. You want to hear from these folks; you need their words of encouragement. But you may be too exhausted to even listen.

You can show your appreciation without picking up the phone. If you have an answering machine, leave an outgoing message like the following, in which you explain how you're doing and that you'll call when you feel up to it. You can tailor the message to more or less information, depending on how discreet you want to be.

> *Hi, this is _____. We thank you for calling, and we very much appreciate your well wishes and concern. As you can understand, we are exhausted from being swamped with appointments and treatments. Your message is very important to us, and we will do our best to get back to you when we're able to take a breather. But if we don't call right away, still know that we are thinking of you and that your support means all the world to us right now. It's good to hear from you!*

PCMS Tool #2.9: Throw a Party

Having a party is another way to say thank-you to the people you have invited into your inner circle of supporters. You may not be in a celebratory mood when you plan it, but you will be once the gathering is in full swing. Perhaps you view a party as one more stressful experience you don't need right now. But if you approach it with the right attitude—and lots of help—it could turn out to be the perfect stress-blaster!

Think of a party as an opportunity to spend time with those you love, no matter what happens next. What you are doing is creating community. And in this particular community, you are the focal point. If you're the type who resists being the center of attention—who feels you aren't worth all the fuss or who says "Yeah, sure, they're fawning over me now that I may be dying"—get over it! You can always fool everyone and live. And

then you can have another party—a victory celebration!

The party itself can be small and intimate—perhaps your immediate family and very closest friends gathered for a Sunday brunch or an afternoon barbecue in the backyard. Or it could be a fancy catered affair, with a buffet and waiters bearing trays of finger foods. You might plan it around a particular event, such as a talent night featuring homegrown entertainment or a (gentle) roast in which participants rib you with funny stories from your checkered past. Of course, they also may lavish great praise on your good deeds.

Try to keep the party upbeat and fun. Sure, it will have its sentimental and emotional moments, but it shouldn't dwell on those. Party favors, plenty of picture taking and videotaping, lots of leftovers, a book for guests to sign—all will ensure that memories linger for weeks and months to come.

Saar and I decided to throw a birthday party for him 8 months after he had been diagnosed with cancer and right after he had been told he was in remission. We made it a black-tie dinner and sent out invitations to about 30 close friends who had been there for us from the start. Saar looked elegant in his tuxedo, even if it sort of swam on him due to his weight loss. I ordered balloons, and we handed out buttons that read "Saar's Supporters."

We asked guests to either prepare short skits, write poems, sing songs, or simply tell a tale or story. We wanted the mood to be upbeat and optimistic. Not that we were going into denial about the facts; not that we wouldn't or couldn't have schmaltzy moments. We just weren't going to let those thoughts and feelings overwhelm us and ruin the celebration of Saar's life—with an emphasis on *life*. We talked about that night often.

Natural Teamwork

This is a time when the company of others who know you well, whom you love and trust, will never be more welcome. While you may have moments when you're too tired to go out, too grumpy to welcome visitors, or too preoccupied to sit through a movie or a play, you will feel energized by the activity. A good conversation—or even a bad one—will draw you out of yourself. It will distract you from worrying about your situation long enough to give you a break from all that's going on. Understand, too, that if you're overwhelmed by the companionship and togetherness, you're allowed to drop out when you need to.

Remember that it's the nature of all living things to support one another. In the fall of each year, wild geese leave Canada and head south for the winter, flying in V formation. As each bird flaps its wings, it creates an updraft for the bird immediately behind it. In this way, a flock can fly farther with greater ease because the geese are helping each other.

When a bird falls out of formation, it feels the drag and resistance of going it alone and rejoins the flock. When the lead bird is tired, he rotates to the back of the flock, and another bird takes his place. All the geese honk to support and encourage the lead bird to keep up the speed.

When one of the flock is sick or wounded and falls out of formation, two geese follow behind to offer protection. They stay with him until he can fly or he dies. Then they move on to catch up with their flock.

We can learn something from this. All of us do better in groups. Offering help seems to come naturally to us. Why refuse the offers that will come from others?

Division of Labor

TASK	WHO WILL DO IT		
	YOU	PERSONAL ADVOCATE	CPA
1. Prepare a script and practice breaking your news.			
2. Tell your immediate family and closest friends.			
3. Tell your boss and co-workers.			
4. Make a list of your supporters.			
5. Make a list of jobs and responsibilities.			
6. Call a meeting of your support team, with your coordinator leading it.			
7. Make a plan for staying in touch with your supporters.			

S T E P   3

UNDERSTAND YOUR DIAGNOSIS

Cancer comes with a steep learning curve. From the moment of your diagnosis, your doctor will be using terms you aren't familiar with and citing statistics you can't compute. Which facts must you have and which can you do without? You need to get up to speed quickly, because you'll be making lots of decisions as you move ahead.

In this chapter, we'll provide information and insight to help interpret your diagnosis. It's important for comparing and choosing treatments, as well as for assembling the best medical team. You'll have a better sense of the research you need to do, the specialists you should look for, and questions you ought to be asking. Understanding your diagnosis may bring out the best in your doctor, too. The two of you can have a more open dialogue about issues that will affect you and your care.

START YOUR CANCER NOTEBOOK

By now, you've amassed enough information that you're ready to create your cancer notebook. It's a tool that you won't want to be without.

Think of your notebook as a living document. You can add to it as you collect information and formulate an action plan. Take time to reread it before every appointment, perhaps while you're sitting in the waiting room. You're more interesting than the celebrities in *People* and *Newsweek*. As your notebook fills up, you may want to pull out and carry with you only those pages relevant to each day's appointments. Put them in your notebook when you return home.

Get a binder with big rings, to allow room for growth. Start by copying and inserting the following worksheets from Steps 1 and 2.

- How Inclusive Are You? A Self-Assessment (page 13)

- Being Inclusive: Identify Your Resistors (page 15)

- Being Inclusive: Take Control of Your Resistors (page 17)

- Being Inclusive: Stop! Reflect! Clarify! (page 20)

- Declaration of Dependence (page 29)

- Use RECE to Communicate Effectively (page 42)

- My Supporters (page 48)

- Support Team Assignments (page 49)

You can photocopy and add other worksheets as you proceed through the steps of the Personal Cancer Management System (PCMS). Be sure to include a notepad or blank sheets of notebook paper, as well as extra pockets for collecting medical records. You can obtain copies of your records, along with lab reports and x-rays, from your various doctors. New federal guidelines guarantee your right to this information. If you ask for these documents at the time of each appointment, you won't need to chase after them later on. Be aware that some doctors and facilities may charge fees for duplication services.

You might want to carry your notebook in a tote bag or briefcase. Then you'll have extra room in case you need it for oversize x-rays or other large materials.

PCMS Tool #3.1: Record Your Medical History

In our experience, it's helpful to have a copy of your medical history with you as you travel to your appointments. Then if any questions arise—about prescriptions or allergies, for example—the answers are right at your fingertips. At the end of the form (opposite page) is space for noting information that doesn't appear elsewhere but seems to come up frequently in your office visits.

Once you've completed this form, you may want to make extra copies for your medical team (which we'll discuss a bit later).

PCMS Tool #3.2: Keep Track

If you're looking at an x-ray or a scan of your cancer, you might not know what to make of the image. A benign growth can appear big,

(continued on page 62)

RECORD YOUR MEDICAL HISTORY

Name_____

Date_____

GENERAL INFORMATION

Age_____ Birth Date_____

Address_____

Home Phone_____ Work Phone_____

Cell/Fax_____

E-mail Address_____

SS#_____

EMPLOYMENT STATUS

Full-Time____ Part-Time_____ School_____ Retired_____ Unemployed_____

Occupation_____

Employer_____

Address_____

Status: Single_____ Married_____ Divorced_____ Widowed_____

Name of Partner/Spouse/Parent_____

Occupation_____

EMERGENCY CONTACT

Name_____ Phone_____

ALLERGIES

Drug Allergies_____

Other Allergies (foods, pollens, etc.)

_____

MEDICAL STATUS

General health before cancer diagnosis

Excellent_____ Good_____ Fair_____ Poor_____

(continued)

RECORD YOUR MEDICAL HISTORY

MEDICATIONS

Prescriptions (include dosages)

_____

_____

_____

_____

Over-the-Counter Drugs and Nutritional Supplements (include dosages)

_____

_____

_____

_____

SCREENING EXAMS

Cholesterol   Date_____

Results_____

Mammogram   Date_____

Results_____

Colonoscopy   Date_____

Results_____

Cardiovascular

Treadmill Test   Date_____   Results_____

Stress Test   Date_____   Results_____

Other

Type_____ Date_____ Results_____

Type_____ Date_____ Results_____

HOSPITALIZATIONS/SURGERIES

Date	Hospital	Diagnosis/Procedure	Doctor

RECORD YOUR MEDICAL HISTORY

CURRENT/RECENT HEALTH CARE PROVIDERS

Name   Dates   Care Provided

_____

_____

_____

_____

PAST MEDICAL CONDITIONS

Childhood Diseases

German Measles_____ Chicken Pox_____ Other_____

Circulatory Disorders

Heart Disease_____ High Blood Pressure_____ Stroke_____ Varicose Veins_____
Phlebitis_____ Clotting Disorder_____ Bleeding Tendencies_____

Other

Diabetes_____ Kidney Trouble_____ Rheumatic Fever_____ Jaundice/Hepatitis_____
Epilepsy_____ Arthritis_____ Colitis_____ Asthma_____
Chronic Fatigue_____ Eating Disorder_____ Cancer_____
Fracture_____ Blood Transfusion_____

FAMILY HISTORY OF CANCER

Name   Relationship   Type of Cancer

_____

_____

_____

_____

NOTES

_____

_____

_____

_____

dark, and ugly, while a malignant one can be invisible to the naked eye—detectable only in the numbers that come back after various tests.

Over the past half century, doctors and researchers have come up with agreed-upon terminology to describe a particular illness and its likely path. These terms, known as parameters, define your particular kind of cancer. All aim at identifying the best treatment and predicting the outcome.

Using the disease parameters, you can determine the speed at which you need to move forward. For instance, if you have a particularly aggressive cancer that is in an advanced stage, your doctor probably will want to begin treatment as soon as possible. This is when you must ask hard questions and get clear answers about timeline and urgency.

Some people feel shy about pushing for answers. Others get angry at themselves when they settle for "We've got to get started," without finding out what would happen if they took time to get a second opinion. With a very aggressive disease, your best bet may be to begin treatment now and get a second opinion along the way. Most often, though, you have a window of opportunity in which you can do research and carefully weigh your options before making decisions.

Here's a rundown of the disease parameters that your doctor will assess.

Type and subtype: These parameters are indicators of the particular tissues that a cancer affects. With kidney cancer, for example, the type is renal cell carcinoma. In other words, the cancer is in the renal (or kidney) tissues. It's possible to further narrow down the classification to subtype, with tests performed by a pathologist. In the case of renal cell carcinoma, the subtype can be clear cell or granular cell—referring to how well differentiated the cells are. The more that's known about your type and subtype of cancer, the better your doctor can match treatment options.

Site: The body part in which a cancer first appears is known as the primary site. Doctors always describe cancer in terms of the primary site, even if it has spread to another body part. If kidney cancer spreads to the lymph nodes, for example, it is still kidney cancer.

The primary site can help determine how a cancer will behave, whether it will spread (metastasize) and where, and what symptoms it may cause. Sometimes the primary site is unknown, in which case your doctor may recommend further testing to help pinpoint it.

Occasionally physicians will attempt to treat a cancer without knowing the primary site. This is done only when they've exhausted all avenues for identifying the site and need to begin treatment without delay.

Stage: Staging refers to how far a cancer has progressed, based on how large the primary tumor is and whether and where it has spread. Depending on the type of cancer, there can be as many as five stages, from 0 to IV. Once you know the stage, you can better understand how advanced your cancer is, how rapidly it is growing, and how much time you have before you must begin treatment.

An early-stage cancer probably will be small and confined to its primary site. It will have a low number. In kidney cancer, stage I tumors are 7 centimeters or smaller in size and limited to the kidney. Late-stage cancers tend to be larger, and they're more likely to have spread to other body parts.

Survival rate: This statistic reflects the odds of surviving for 5 years after diagnosis, based on the stage of cancer. Stage I kidney cancer has a survival rate of 70 percent. For some people, this information is encouraging; for others, it is not. You might want to think carefully before inquiring about the survival rate for your particular cancer, perhaps discussing it with your doctor, your personal advocate, or your family members.

Risk factors: Since you already know you have cancer, the risk factors—such as age, gender, medical history, genetic history, and environment—may seem irrelevant. But if your cancer has a genetic component, you may want to inform your children. Then they can work with their doctors to decide whether they should undergo early screening or consider other preventive measures. Keep in mind that while genetics plays a role in some cancers (such as breast and pancreatic cancers), it doesn't mean that your children are certain to get the disease, too.

As you gather information about your particular cancer, you can use the chart on page 64 to take notes. We've included space to write down which physicians you've consulted and which tests you've undergone. This way, all the information relevant to your diagnosis is in one place.

Don't Forget to Write!

You're certain that you'll remember what Dr. X or Dr. Y said during your appointment. You couldn't help but give your full attention to what was being said. Yet research shows that people forget about 80 percent of the information from their doctors' visits soon after leaving the office. The more critical and stressful the discussion, the more quickly they forget.

So on your way out, stop for a moment—in the waiting room, in the building lobby or coffee shop, or at least in the car—to write down what your doctor said. Read it over with a family member or friend when you get home. Better yet, take someone with you to jot down notes while you focus on what your doctor is saying.

Through this process, you likely will think of follow-up questions or points for further discussion with your doctor. You also may find information that requires clarification. Make a list so you remember for your next appointment. If it can't wait, call your doctor that day or the next, before the urgency fades.

INVESTIGATE YOUR TREATMENT OPTIONS

Once you know the particulars of your kind of cancer, you can launch a more targeted search of your treatment options. As you'll discover, you have many options to consider. New therapies and techniques are being developed and tested all the time. Your job—with the help of your personal advocate and perhaps your cancer patient advocate—is to find out as much as possible about what's out there and which approach offers the best prospect of success for you.

Your doctor probably discussed some treatments with you at the time of diagnosis. If

PCMS Tool #3.2

KEEP TRACK My Cancer Profile

TYPE AND SUBTYPE	
SITE	
STAGE	
SURVIVAL RATE	
RISK FACTORS	
CONSULTATIONS	
TESTS/RESULTS	

you seek out a second opinion—an interesting and sometimes sensitive process that we'll discuss in Step 4 (page 96)—you may come away with more options. Your own research could turn up other possibilities that neither doctor mentioned.

As you move forward with treatment, you may choose to make adjustments—trying new approaches that emerge from clinical trials, eliminating those with side effects or long-term effects that undermine quality of life, or possibly integrating complementary and alternative medicine with conventional therapies. So though you may gather more information than you can use right away, just keep it. It may come in handy later on.

To help guide your search for treatments, we've mapped out a seven-step action plan for you.

1. Cast a Wide Net

In the information-gathering stage, any and all treatments should get fair consideration. Don't rule out anything just yet. What might not appeal to you now may turn out to be your best option.

Draw on the collective wisdom of your family physician and local oncologists, as well as research by medical oncologists—national experts who study your particular type of cancer. (We'll talk more about the various oncology specialists a bit later.) Practitioners of complementary and alternative therapies can offer suggestions, as can the members of your support team.

Of course, doing this research will take time—time you may not feel you have. If you

haven't done so already, this is when you should ask your doctor hard questions about how quickly you need to begin treatment. You need a clear sense of the time frame so you can plan your search strategy.

Keep in mind that once you know the specifics of your cancer, you probably can collect treatment information via phone and e-mail consultations rather than in-person office visits. Going the virtual route can be especially helpful for getting input from cancer experts whose practices are clear across the country.

2. Survey Conventional Standardized Treatments

The phrase "conventional standardized treatment" usually refers to a treatment regimen that specifies dosage, schedule, and duration. While they may be modified for individual patients, these regimens have been standardized under the clinical practice guidelines of the American Society of Clinical Oncology, surgical and radiation oncology groups, and other relevant organizations. The specific drugs, devices, and techniques used in these regimens have been approved by the US Food and Drug Administration (FDA).

On the other hand, a *protocol* is a clinical trial, although these days the word may pop up in everyday conversation to describe any treatment plan. A protocol tells us what a study will do, how many people will be participating, who is eligible, which drugs or interventions will be used, and what will be learned. If you are receiving a protocol, the treatment has reached the stage of being safe for humans, but it hasn't been approved by the FDA.

With these definitions in mind, let's review the conventional standardized treatments and protocols that you likely will encounter in your research.

Chemotherapy: This involves the intravenous injection and/or infusion of one or more drugs into the bloodstream through a shunt implanted in the arm or clavicle (collarbone). Essentially, these drugs poison the cancer. Depending on whether or not a chemo "cocktail" uses drugs currently in clinical trials or adds a new drug to an old "recipe," it may qualify as a conventional standardized treatment or a protocol. Ask your doctor to specify the ingredients in the cocktail you'd be getting. Each treatment regimen or protocol has its own success rate and its own side effects. Ask what they are and what they mean for you.

Usually chemotherapy requires a series of visits to a treatment center—for instance, twice a week for two periods of 3 weeks, with a week off in between. Each visit can last from 1 to several hours. The series is repeated as needed. Some hospitals or cancer centers prefer to administer chemotherapy on an inpatient basis, while others offer it as an outpatient service.

Some newer chemotherapies such as imatinib (Gleevec) and thalidomide can be taken orally. Others are administered by a battery-powered pack worn on the waist, which means you can stay mobile during treatment.

Cryosurgery: This treatment technique directly attacks a tumor by freezing the cancer cells.

Radiation therapy: More than half of all people who have cancer receive radiation therapy. This treatment regimen targets specific areas of the body where the cancer appears to be concentrating. X-ray waves or radio waves either destroy cancer cells or damage them so badly that they can't multiply.

Radiation therapy takes two forms.

- *Brachytherapy,* or internal therapy, involves implanting a radioactive source inside the body near the cancerous growth.

- *External beam radiation,* or teletherapy, directs radiation from an outside source into the body. A machine positioned several feet from the patient strikes the target area with radiation. Recent advances in radiation oncology—including gamma knife, cyber knife, intensity modulated radiation therapy (IMRT), and proton therapy—offer more precise methods of reaching the cancer. Of these techniques, proton therapy uses a proton particle beam, while the rest rely on photons. Typically, external beam radiation is administered 5 days a week for a period of several weeks.

Surgery: The earliest form of modern cancer therapy, surgery involves cutting out a malignant tumor before it spreads or metastasizes. A number of surgical procedures are available, each for a particular type of cancer. Which one a doctor recommends will vary according to the type and stage of cancer, the health and tolerance of the patient, and other individual factors.

PCMS Tool #3.3: Compare Treatments

Gathering information about your treatment options will take you into unfamiliar territory. You may need help keeping track of all the details. The tool on page 68 should come in handy. It can accommodate three treatments. Feel free to make more copies if necessary, as you collect more data.

As you'll notice, we've included space for notes about risks and side effects. We believe that both are critical to your consideration of your treatment options, because they can have a significant impact on your quality of life. For example, cancer patients who undergo chemotherapy often report fatigue, nausea, pain, and sleep problems. Many experience hair loss and weight loss, which affects their body image. Chemotherapy also opens the door to opportunistic conditions such as shingles and thrush. The question for you is, will you be able to tolerate these side effects—not just physically but also psychologically?

We're not suggesting that you discount a treatment because the potential side effects trouble you. Rather, you should discuss them with your doctor—who may address your concerns by offering alternatives for administering the treatment. For example, if you'll be getting chemotherapy, your doctor may adjust your schedule so you have more recovery days between treatments. Your doctor might know of complementary and alternative therapies that can help minimize side effects. Or you could try a treatment for a while, to see how you feel.

3. Explore Cutting-Edge Medicine

All medications—whether for cancer or for another disease—start out in a laboratory, where they must undergo rigorous scientific study. Once a particular medication crosses critical research hurdles and is deemed safe and beneficial, it's ready for testing in humans. This testing is known as a clinical trial.

Thousands of clinical trials are under way in the United States and all over the world. The National Cancer Institute is sponsoring research on more than 250 cancer agents. In clinical trials for cancer agents, the research teams consist of specialists from many fields, including research medical oncologists who are national experts in specific cancers. They carefully design and monitor the trials to ensure accurate outcomes.

In the case of cancer, not all clinical trials are for the purpose of finding a new treatment. Some aim at prevention; others intend to extend life or improve quality of life, such as those for pain management. Once a cancer agent is put in a clinical trial, it becomes available to the medical community and to those patients who are most likely to benefit from the agent and the protocol.

As you gather preliminary information about the treatment options for your type of cancer, be sure to look into relevant clinical trials and their protocols. Interviewing the experts who've developed these protocols could provide leads on cancer agents that are awaiting testing or that already are available for use. Even if you have no interest in participating in a clinical trial, you'll gain knowledge

(continued on page 70)

PCMS Tool #3.3 (Sample)

COMPARE TREATMENTS

DIAGNOSIS	Non-Hodgkin's lymphoma		
	OPTION #1	OPTION #2	OPTION #3
TREATMENT	Chemotherapy/ Rituxan + CHOP	Chemotherapy/ Rituxan + CHOP; radiation	
FREQUENCY	One cycle every 6 weeks; 6 cycles total	Chemotherapy: once every 3 weeks for six cycles; radiation: 5 times per week for 6 weeks	
BENEFITS	Possible total remission	Possible total remission	
RISKS	Immuno-suppression	Immuno-suppression	
SIDE EFFECTS	Nausea and fatigue	Nausea and fatigue	
SUCCESS RATE	Long-term survival: 40–60%	Long-term survival: 60–70%	
COST	Full insurance coverage	Full insurance coverage	
YOUR DECISION (circle one)	Yes No More research	Yes No More research	

COMPARE TREATMENTS

DIAGNOSIS			
	OPTION #1	OPTION #2	OPTION #3
TREATMENT			
FREQUENCY			
BENEFITS			
RISKS			
SIDE EFFECTS			
SUCCESS RATE			
COST			
YOUR DECISION (circle one)	Yes No More research	Yes No More research	

69

about the most advanced treatments, which you then can use as a benchmark for comparing your other options. Plus, your findings will feed the dialogue between you and your doctor, helping to build collaboration and trust between the two of you.

If you've brought a cancer patient advocate into your support team, this person can help identify clinical trials and experimental protocols on your behalf. You also might check the following Web sites.

- http://med.stanford.edu
- www.cancer.gov
- www.cancercare.org
- www.cancernet.nci.nih.gov/trials
- www.cancertrialshelp.org
- www.clinicaltrials.gov
- www.veritasmedicine.com/index.cfm
- www.centerwatch.com
- www.acurian.com/nws_home_page.jsp

Following are brief descriptions of several cancer agents that are in clinical trials as of this writing. Our list is not inclusive, but it will give you some idea of what you might find in your search.

Assay-directed cancer therapy: This form of chemotherapy grew from the idea that each cancer patient is unique, so therefore cancer treatment must be customized to the patient in order to be effective. Assay-directed cancer therapy involves harvesting diseased tissue through surgery, then subjecting it to a procedure known as ex vivo apoptotic assay. Essentially, the tissue is injected with various chemotherapy drugs to see which one it is

most sensitive to. That will be the drug with the greatest potential to kill the cancer. Conversely, other drugs to which the cancer might be resistant can be ruled out.

Assay-directed cancer therapy remains in an experimental stage. You can find further information about this therapy by visiting the Web sites of the following research facilities.

- Genzyme Genetics: www.genzyme genetics.com
- Oncotech: www.oncotech.com
- Precision Therapeutics: www.precision therapeutics.com
- Rational Therapeutics: www. rational-t.com
- Weisenthal Cancer Group: www.weisenthal.org

Chemoprevention: This involves the use of natural or synthetic agents to reduce the risk of recurrence in people who've already had cancer, as well as to protect those who've never had the disease. Perhaps the best-known chemopreventives are tamoxifen (Nolvadex) and raloxifene (Evista), which belong to a class of drugs known as selective estrogen receptor modulators (SERMs). Taken orally, these drugs can help prevent recurrence of breast cancer. Another chemopreventive is thalidomide, which helps maintain cancer remission by acting as an antiangiogenesis agent. In other words, it chokes off the blood supply to a developing tumor.

More chemopreventive drugs are in clinical trials. For example, researchers are studying whether sulindac (Clinoril)—alone or in combination with other drugs—can prevent colon cancer in people who are at high risk for the disease.

For the latest information on chemopreventive agents, visit the Web site for the National Cancer Institute's Chemopreventive Agent Development Research Group: www.cancer.gov/prevention/cadrg.

Gene therapy: In one especially active area of cancer research, scientists are performing gene expression profiles on cancerous tissue. Their goal is to determine how particular chemotherapy drugs affect particular gene clusters. Eventually, this research might lead to a sort of early warning system, enabling doctors to predict when a localized cancer will metastasize and therefore require treatment sooner rather than later.

One test based on gene therapy research already is available. Known as the oncotype DX assay for node-negative estrogen receptor-positive disease, it uses breast tumor tissue to identify and analyze 16 different cancer genes and five reference genes. The results indicate whether a woman with breast cancer is at low or high risk for recurrence. If she's at low risk, hormone therapy may be sufficient; if she's at high risk, chemotherapy followed by hormone therapy may prove more helpful.

PCMS Tool #3.4: Compare Clinical Trials

Even once you narrow your search to your type of cancer, you probably will find more information on clinical trials than will fit in the chart on page 73. Streamline the data by identifying the highlights, then personalizing

it as much as possible. Note your strengths and liabilities in terms of eligibility. With regard to the phase of the trial, use the following key.

I: The first phase to be tried on human subjects

II: The phase that valuates details such as benefits and safe dosage

III: The final phase leading to approval or nonapproval by the FDA

Even though you're recording the trial information in the chart, always print the descriptions from the Web sites. That way it's handy should you need it for further reference.

4. Think Long-Term

With so many decisions before you, this may not seem like the time to be thinking about the future. But the fact is, you can pursue measures now that may save your life later. You may change your course of treatment if your first regimen doesn't produce the results that you and your doctor expect. Or you may switch to a maintenance regimen once your treatment ends. Either route may require some advance planning on your part, especially if you'll need to meet certain eligibility requirements.

Medical research is advancing at a faster rate than ever. Therapies that are entering the research pipeline now might be ready for clinical trial as you're ready to try them. Your personal advocate or cancer patient advocate can stay on top of these developments, so you can concentrate on your treatment and recovery.

71

(continued on page 74)

PCMS Tool #3.4 (Sample)

COMPARE CLINICAL TRIALS

DIAGNOSIS	Non-Hodgkin's lymphoma		
	OPTION #1	**OPTION #2**	**OPTION #3**
SOURCE	Clinicaltrials.gov	National Institutes of Health site	
TITLE	Combo chemo > radiation	# ID03-0001 lymphoma	
PHYSICIAN	N/A	Pro, Barbara	
SPONSOR	German Hi-Grade NHL Study Center	Genta Inc.	
PURPOSE	Evaluate certain drugs	Evaluate gallium nitrate	
TREATMENT OR INTERVENTION	5 drugs, including prednisone, every 3 weeks for 6 cycles; radiation 5 times per week for 4 weeks; other therapies	Every 3 weeks for 1 year, then every 3 months; at M.D. Anderson	
PHASE (I, II, OR III)	III	II	
OBJECTIVES	Compare drugs and long-term effects	Test safety of drug	
GUIDELINES	Randomly assigned to one of two different protocols	Outpatient	
ELIGIBILITY • DISEASE CHARACTERISTICS	Previously untreated. No more than 25% disease involvement	Prior treatment OK Ø Allograft Ø Corticosteroids	
• PATIENT CHARACTERISTICS	Ages 18–60 Ø Second cancer Correct platelet counts	Ø Pregnancy Ø Hepatitis	
OTHER SPECS	HIV negative Ø Pregnancy	See list	
YOUR DECISION (CIRCLE ONE)	(Yes) No More research	Yes (No) More research	
CONTACT	See list on printout		

COMPARE CLINICAL TRIALS

DIAGNOSIS			
	OPTION #1	OPTION #2	OPTION #3
SOURCE			
TITLE			
PHYSICIAN			
SPONSOR			
PURPOSE			
TREATMENT OR INTERVENTION			
PHASE (I, II, OR III)			
OBJECTIVES			
GUIDELINES			
ELIGIBILITY • DISEASE CHARACTERISTICS			
• PATIENT CHARACTERISTICS			
OTHER SPECS			
YOUR DECISION (CIRCLE ONE)	Yes No More research	Yes No More research	
CONTACT			

73

We realize that thinking so far in advance isn't for everyone, especially when you're facing more immediate decisions about your treatment. But if you want this sort of information now, start by talking to your doctor about what's next. Do your homework on the Internet. Consult cancer survivors. And be open to what you find!

To get a head start on your search, you might want to look into the following therapies, which either are in development or may call for advance planning.

Bone marrow/stem cell transplants: Oncologists sometimes recommend transplants in an effort to enhance the effectiveness of treatment or to extend remission. Prior to the procedure, patients usually receive an extra round of high-dose chemotherapy to eliminate as much of the cancer as possible.

You may be most familiar with bone marrow transplants, in which blood-building cells are drawn from either the patient's or a donor's marrow and infused into the patient's blood supply. The body uses these fresh cells to generate its own healthy blood and immune cells. Stem cell transplants work in a similar fashion. Immature blood cells are filtered and stimulated with growth factors to produce stem cells, which are then infused into the bloodstream to generate healthy cells.

When a patient uses his or her own blood cells for a transplant procedure, it's known as an autologous transplant. This procedure has become much safer in recent years, though it still carries some risk. In an allogenic transplant, the blood cells come from a donor. Allogenic transplants carry a higher risk of host versus graft disease, since the host—your

body—must adjust to the foreign matter that has been "grafted" into it.

If this treatment option is appropriate for your type of cancer, you need to know what kind of donor would be eligible and who in your family might be a suitable candidate, or whether you must go to a donor bank. This process takes time, and it involves sensitive discussions with family members.

Vaccine therapy: When you hear the word *vaccine,* you probably think of the injections that protect against diseases such as measles in children and flu in adults. Vaccines work by introducing just enough of the disease-causing agent into the body to evoke an immune response, thereby building resistance to the agent.

Scientists are developing vaccines to protect against recurrences of breast cancer, prostate cancer, lymphoma, and multiple myeloma. Rather than the usual one-size-fits-all inoculation that offers equal protection to everyone, cancer vaccines combine a protein that's unique to a patient's diseased tissue with dendritic cells. These cells police the body, gobbling up suspect proteins while displaying markers for the diseased tissue on their surface. This alerts other immune cells known as killer T cells that an enemy is present and they need to destroy it.

The department of oncology at Stanford University—which administers the Stanford Vaccine Program—and the Comprehensive Cancer Center at St. Vincent's Hospital in New York City are among several facilities to offer experimental vaccines to eligible multiple myeloma patients who have harvested diseased tissue. The vaccines are given in combination with conventional therapies following various research protocols, such as before, during, or after transplants. The objective of these particular protocols is to prevent cancer recurrence.

Other innovations in vaccine therapy may emerge just as you reach a critical juncture in your treatment. For example, Stanford Hospital and Clinics and its partner hospitals are experimenting with the combination of vaccines and transplants to improve the outcome of lymphoma treatment.

The Web site www.clinicaltrials.gov lists more than 100 clinical trials (as of this writing) that are actively recruiting patients with various types of cancer for vaccine therapy. To qualify for one of these trials, *you must harvest and bank your own diseased tissue before treatment destroys it.* So even if you have no intention of trying vaccine therapy at present, you may want to talk with your doctor about harvesting tissue, just in case you change your mind.

Maintenance regimens: Once you've outwitted cancer by going into remission, your next task will be to outwit its return. The objective of a maintenance regimen is to at least hold the status quo—for example, preserving remission and/or managing any residual disease. While the jury is out on the effectiveness of these programs, many experts believe that they improve a patient's odds of extending remission.

Transplants and vaccines could qualify as maintenance regimens, in the sense that they keep cancer at bay after another treatment wipes it out. A more standard regimen is to follow high-dose chemotherapy with alpha interferon, a drug that inhibits the spread of cancer cells in hairy cell leukemia, follicular lymphoma, and multiple myeloma, among other cancers. In studies, cancer patients who receive this maintenance protocol remain in remission far longer than patients who don't. At certain doses, alpha-interferon can cause side effects such as depression, hallucinations, and psychoses, so quality of life is an important consideration here.

Another maintenance regimen, molecularly targeted therapy, blocks the growth and spread of cancer by interfering with specific molecules on a tumor cell's surface. Among the drugs approved by the FDA for this purpose are erlotinib (Tarceva) and Erbitux, for non-small-cell lung and colorectal cancers; and bevacizumab (Avastin), for colorectal cancer.

If you think you might be interested in a maintenance regimen, it's best to inform your doctor at the outset of treatment. That way, your doctor can determine your eligibility for such a program well in advance of your needing it. The sooner you get those wheels in motion, the better. Newer maintenance regimens are in the pipeline now, so watch for them. And since existing regimens can fall out of favor, pay attention for that news, too.

In addition to the earlier listing of Web sites for clinical trials, all of the following are good resources for information on maintenance regimens.

- Call the National Cancer Institute's Cancer Information Services hotline (800-422-6237). It maintains a comprehensive computerized database for cancer diagnosis, treatment, and prevention. You'll get a printout of relevant trials within a five- to six-state radius of your home.

- Contact local cancer centers or the department of oncology at a local hospital. Ask to speak with a clinical research nurse or protocol coordinator responsible for recruiting study volunteers.

- Consult a national expert in your type of cancer. That person may be working on one of the protocols you've read about.

- Inquire with your local chapter of the American Cancer Society, as well as local cancer patient support groups. They may be aware of open clinical trials in your area.

- Contact the pharmaceutical company that developed the protocol you're interested in. The *Physicians' Desk Reference* lists addresses and phone numbers for all prescription drug manufacturers. You can look up this information online at www.pdr.net. You also might check www.phrma.org/newmedicines/, an industry-sponsored site that provides profiles of drugs in development.

5. Take an Integrative Approach

Integrative medicine is a newish term that applies to the combination of conventional treatment methods with complementary and alternative medicine (CAM). Though these therapies can't cure cancer, they can help you cope with the physical and psychological effects of the disease. For this reason, you may

want to explore your CAM options early on, with the prospect of adding one or more to your treatment plan.

Over the last 30 years, CAM has grown in popularity and acceptance, as scientific research confirms its therapeutic value. Beyond relieving physical side effects such as pain, fatigue, and nausea, CAM therapies appear especially helpful in offsetting the stress, anxiety, and depression that frequently accompany cancer and its treatment. These psychological side effects trigger excess production of the hormones norepinephrine and cortisol, which weaken the immune system and allow more opportunistic diseases to move in. This debilitates patients and threatens their physical and emotional ability to handle aggressive treatment.

Research bears out the ability of some CAM therapies to bolster the immune system. With stronger immune function, you'll be better able to tolerate the side effects of chemotherapy or radiation without reducing dosage or suspending treatment. Many cancer patients have reported that acupuncture and massage dramatically reduce the nausea and fatigue that often follow chemotherapy. Likewise, disciplines such as yoga, meditation, and energy healing may help reduce the mental and emotional stress of the disease.

We'll discuss CAM at length in Step 6 (page 131). Here are brief descriptions of a number of CAM professions, so you can get some sense of what's available to you.

- *Acupuncturists* adhere to the traditional Chinese medicine principle that energy flows along pathways called meridians.

By inserting fine sterile needles along the meridians, acupuncturists can help relieve the nausea associated with chemotherapy, as well as fatigue, lower back pain, headache, and anxiety.

- *Biofeedback trainers* provide instruction in controlling bodily functions such as breathing and blood pressure.

- *Chiropractors* can help manage pain by releasing blockages along the nerve bundles inside the spinal cord.

- *Clergy* offer spiritual support through prayer and other faith-based practices.

- *Cognitive rehabilitation therapists* can help correct the effects of chemotherapy on mental function.

- *Dance and music therapists* tap into the healing influence of rhythm, similar to the Baby Einstein products that support brain development in infants.

- *Energy healing therapists* practice the transfer of energy from one person to another. Known in scientific circles as psychoneuroimmunology, this practice currently is the subject of research at UCLA's Semel Institute for Neuroscience and Human Behavior.

- *Herbalists* recommend herbal supplements to improve immune function and alleviate the side effects of cancer treatment.

- *Hypnotherapists* use hypnosis to help manage stress, relieve pain, and reduce nausea.

- *Massage therapists* use physical manipulation to stimulate blood flow and lymphatic circulation, which can improve sleep and minimize side effects.

- *Meditation instructors* use breath and visual imagery to tap the therapeutic power of the mind and relax the body.

- *Nutritionists* develop special diets for cancer patients, especially to offset the rapid weight loss that may occur during treatment.

- *Psycho-oncologists* are psychiatrists, psychologists, social workers, counselors, and other health professionals who have received specific training to assist cancer patients and their loved ones. Psychiatrists who practice this interdisciplinary specialty also offer medication management for physical and psychological side effects.

- *Yoga instructors* teach breathing techniques and poses that can help neutralize and eliminate the toxins that can accumulate in fatty tissues during cancer treatment. Yoga has proven effective for reducing stress as well.

We suggest putting together a short list of the CAM practitioners you may want to consult before or during your treatment. Of course, you are not obligated to try CAM if you don't want to. But rather than rely on last-minute improvisations when your energy and focus are at their lowest, having a list helps keep your CAM options available for when you may need them. Be sure to talk with your doctor before adding any CAM therapy to your treatment plan.

For more information on CAM as well as specific disciplines, visit nccam.nih.gov. It's the Web site of the National Center for Complementary and Alternative Medicine, established in 1998 by the National Institutes of Health.

6. Talk to Survivors

Through the course of your research into treatment options, you'll encounter many kinds of cancer experts. Not all of them will have medical degrees. You may uncover the information that changes your life—and gain a lot of support in the process—by talking to cancer survivors and their families. These people have already been down the path that you're just starting and so can be excellent resources.

Organizations such as the R.A. Bloch Cancer Foundation (www.blochcancer.org) and the National Coalition for Cancer Survivorship (www.canceradvocacy.org) can connect you with survivors who had the same type of cancer that you do. Whether you go through these Web sites or seek out people on your own, it's smart to know in advance what questions you want to ask. Use the following as jumping-off points for your conversation.

- What are the two most important things you can tell me?

- What would you have done differently?

- Did you pursue any cutting-edge treatments? Which ones? Were they helpful?

- Did you try any CAM therapies? Which ones? Were they helpful?

7. Schedule an Appointment with Your Doctor

Once you've scoured the available resources for treatment options, it's time to meet with your doctor to review your findings. Take printouts or photocopies of relevant information to your appointment, so you have them for reference. This is a good opportunity not only to get your doctor's opinion on treatment but also to assess his or her flexibility and openness to your input. It's important for you to feel comfortable relating to your doctor as a partner or collaborator, not a superior.

All of us have a learned tendency to treat doctors with a degree of reverence. The fact is, they're service providers. If you're not confident that your doctor will give you the time, attention, and respect to mutually agree upon a course of treatment, then you need to seriously consider moving on to someone else.

When you meet with your doctor, you can open the conversation by saying, "I've been reading about my disease, and I've found several sources that suggest various treatments. I'm hoping that you can help me sort out my options." Then ask these questions, or substitute some of your own that cover the same ground.

Can you discuss and explain these options? Your doctor may or may not be familiar with the materials you bring in. Notice the response to your proactive efforts and whether he or she is receptive to them.

What is the success rate of the treatment you recommend? How does it compare with others? Your doctor may favor a standard treatment regimen for your cancer even though another therapy offers better odds. Conversely, some innovative treatments may seem to offer hope, but their effectiveness in stopping cancer growth falls short of expectations.

Does the success rate apply to my particular situation, considering my age, medical history, and general health, and the type and stage of my cancer? A preexisting condition such as heart disease or diabetes may disqualify you from certain chemotherapy or radiation treatments. This is why it's so important to be very clear about your medical history and your current health status.

What are the known side effects of this treatment? Very aggressive protocols often have side effects that can undermine your quality of life. You need to consider this when weighing your options.

Which treatments will my insurance pay for? Though you shouldn't use this as the sole basis for your treatment decisions, it certainly will be an influencing factor. Keep in mind that experimental cancer protocols—which often are excluded from health coverage—may cost little or nothing anyway, since they're funded through grants. Be sure to check with your insurance company as well.

If I choose a treatment that you haven't overseen before, must I travel to the cancer center where the national expert in this protocol practices? Or can you administer it here? In most cases, the "recipes" for experimental cancer protocols developed by national experts have been published in medical journals and can be replicated by local physicians.

After reading about Dr. X's research into my type of cancer, I'd like to meet with him in person or talk with him by phone. Would you be able to schedule an appointment on my behalf? If I talk with him by phone, do you want to participate in the call? Some national experts will recommend or require an in-person consultation before rendering an opinion. With others, a phone call will suffice. Having your doctor participate in the call might be helpful. Your doctor's willingness to coordinate this conversation can be a good indicator of the kind of partnership the two of you will have.

ASSEMBLE YOUR MEDICAL TEAM

Cancer is a journey—a quest, really—for the right combination of doctors and treatments to make you well. It likely began with your primary care physician, who referred you to an oncologist for testing. After reviewing the test results, the oncologist confirmed your diagnosis and made initial recommendations for treatment. Your next step is to open up the dialogue to other specialists from a variety of disciplines, with the goal of putting together your medical team.

The skills and strategies that you employed to assemble your support team should come in handy here. Now more than ever, you need to be proactive. Don't hesitate to solicit the opinions of your personal advocate, your cancer patient advocate (if you have one), and other members of your support team in handpicking the professionals who will best serve you. You also might wish to seek referrals from national medical centers such as Massachusetts General Hospital, Memorial Sloan-Kettering Cancer Center,

Johns Hopkins University, Cleveland Clinic, M.D. Anderson Cancer Center, and Dana-Farber/Partners CancerCare.

Though we've said it many times before, it bears repeating here: When assessing the candidates for your medical team, your comfort level should count for just as much as their medical expertise. Research proves that when patients choose doctors with whom they're comfortable, they're more likely to build trusting, productive partnerships. As a result, they feel more capable and more in control of their situations, and they're better able to tolerate treatment. This translates to better quality of life and better outcomes.

Through this process, you may find another oncologist whom you'd like to have oversee your care. Or you may stay with the same one that your primary care physician first recommended, feeling confident that you've made the best choice. Your primary care physician may play a less prominent role moving forward, but hopefully will remain involved as a coach and consultant. After all, this physician knows more about your medical history and health status than anyone—and can provide invaluable guidance as you navigate the cancer process.

The Role of Oncologist

As your medical team takes shape, you may bring onboard not one but several oncologists. Within the realm of oncology are multiple subspecialties, each of which fills a specific role on the cancer treatment continuum. Though they work in the same field of medicine, they won't necessarily share the same view of your particular cancer. That's not a bad thing. Their different philosophies and methodologies will help point you to your full range of treatment options, so you can make informed decisions.

Diagnostic oncologists. The first link in the oncology chain of care is the diagnostic oncologist, who can pinpoint the particulars of a cancer. As an example, let's suppose that a woman has found a lump in her breast. Her primary care physician may refer her to a diagnostic breast oncologist for a complete breast examination, which would include a physical breast exam, a mammogram, and probably an ultrasound. Should these screenings confirm the presence of a lump, the oncologist would be able to gather more information about it via a fine or core needle biopsy or, if necessary, a stereotactic (noninvasive) biopsy. Any of these could rule out a more invasive biopsy procedure. Other suspected cancers may require a radiologic procedure such as an MRI or a CT, PET, or CT/PET scan.

Surgical oncologists. Once the diagnostic oncologist finds a cancer, the surgical oncologist will get rid of it via a surgical procedure. Most of these surgeons specialize in general categories of cancer—such as a surgical gynecological oncologist, who concentrates on women's cancers. Some surgeons narrow their focus to specific types of cancer, such as breast cancer.

Treating medical oncologists. A patient requiring further treatment after surgery may be referred by the surgical oncologist to a treating medical oncologist for chemotherapy. Actually, you may have one of these oncologists on your medical team even if you don't undergo surgery. The treating medical oncologist sees patients on a regular basis, administering treatment and managing side effects. Ideally, it's a local physician, so the patient can stay close to home and to loved ones.

To find a treating medical oncologist who's skilled in administering a particular chemotherapy protocol, your best bet may be to ask the national expert who developed it. You also might look for someone who, though perhaps not familiar with the protocol, has a special interest in treating your type of cancer.

Radiation oncologists. Radiation oncologists fill essentially the same role as treating medical oncologists, only they specialize in radiation therapy. Modern radiation protocols can contribute to cure, in addition to serving as a palliative measure.

Research medical oncologists. Unlike their colleagues, research medical oncologists see patients primarily in the course of carrying out experimental protocols. Their goal is to find cures for specific types of cancer, as well as therapeutic measures that can prolong life or enhance quality of life. Most research medical oncologists are affiliated with university hospitals or national cancer centers.

PCMS Tool #3.5: Record Contact Information

At the core of your medical team will be your treating oncologist. As discussed above, this may be a surgical oncologist, a medical oncologist, or a radiation oncologist. Depending on the particulars of your illness, you may end up collaborating with all three. Be-

yond that, we suggest finding a national expert and a research oncologist who specialize in your cancer. They will serve as consultants, while your treating oncologist is responsible for hands-on treatment. You can build around this core as you wish, until you have a team that collectively can attend to all aspects of your care.

As you talk with these various physicians and find other health professionals who seem like good candidates for your medical team, use the chart on page 82 to keep track of their contact information. It's better to make these notes now than later, when you may not be up to it. Feel free to condense your list as you go along, until your team is in place.

Remember, the goal of all this homework is to cull those cancer experts who are the best matches for you. This means they have the knowledge to help you make informed treatment decisions, as well as the "bedside manner" to support and encourage you along the way. Proximity matters, too: In the ideal scenario, you can find a treating oncologist close by, with a national expert available as necessary.

PCMS Tool #3.6: Diagram Your Medical Team

As you choose your medical team, write each person's name in the appropriate space of the chart on page 83. Add circles as necessary to reflect the composition of your team. And pay attention to those arrows. The purpose here is to make sure that lines of communication remain open among all the team members.

PHYSICIAN CONTACTS

	CONTACT INFO	ADDITIONAL NOTES
NAME: SPECIALTY:	Phone: Fax: Address: E-mail:	
NAME: SPECIALTY:	Phone: Fax: Address: E-mail:	
NAME: SPECIALTY:	Phone: Fax: Address: E-mail:	
NAME: SPECIALTY:	Phone: Fax: Address: E-mail:	
NAME: SPECIALTY:	Phone: Fax: Address: E-mail:	
NAME: SPECIALTY:	Phone: Fax: Address: E-mail:	
NAME: SPECIALTY:	Phone: Fax: Address: E-mail:	

DIAGRAM YOUR MEDICAL TEAM

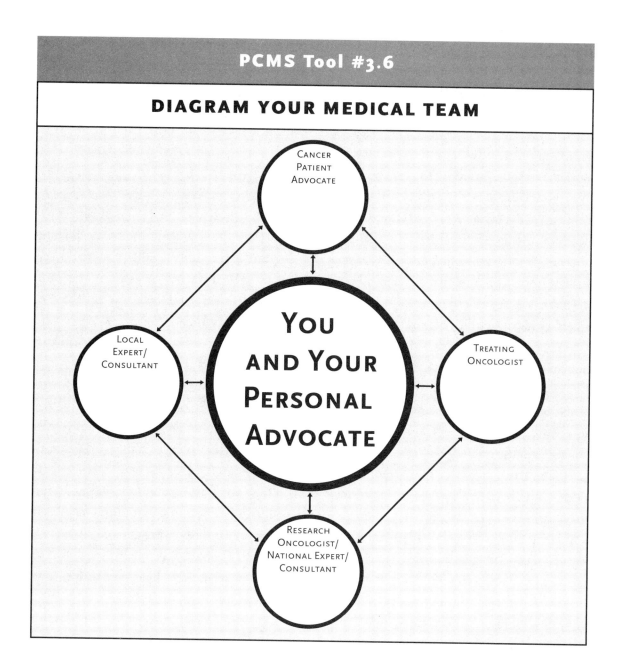

You'll notice that we've included both a local and a national expert in the diagram. If you happen to live in a major metropolitan area, you may be fortunate enough to find someone nearby who's working on a treatment protocol for your type of cancer. You may be able to schedule an in-person consultation.

THE PATIENT-DOCTOR PARTNERSHIP

Cultivating positive, productive relationships among all the members of your medical team—and especially between you and your treating oncologist—won't happen by sheer willpower. It takes work. But it's worth the effort. After all, your medical team is fighting for your life. The more everyone trusts and respects each other, the more open the communication can be.

Once you've done the heavy lifting of assembling your medical team, you may feel the urge to sit back and let the experts determine your course of treatment. Perhaps your resistors will kick in, as you wrestle with the notion of being on equal footing with your doctors. Just because one person has certain academic or professional expertise, that doesn't make the other less equal—especially when it's his or her life that's at stake.

What you're aiming for, ideally, is a relationship that's not so much equal as equitable. In other words, by virtue of bringing different but valuable knowledge and experience to the table, both patient and doctor have equal say in the ensuing dialogue.

If you aren't proactive now, over time the interaction between you and your doctor may come to resemble one of submissive child and powerful parent—with you not wanting to risk displeasing or otherwise alienating your doctor. So you may agree to what you subconsciously believe is not in your best interest. Next thing you know, you're anxious and angry with yourself. That kind of stress can undermine the effectiveness of your treatment, not to mention your quality of life.

When you are proactive, you demonstrate your commitment to the patient/doctor partnership by making it a priority. As a social being, your doctor almost always will reciprocate. In effect, being proactive energizes the connection between the two of you. The art of medicine lies in this connection—doctors knowing their patients well enough to understand intuitively the needs of each one, and patients feeling able to build the kind of trust necessary to be open with their doctors.

It's All about Teamwork

Saar and I always believed that our cancer patients were the drivers in their care, making decisions that would take them to their destination—defeating an overwhelming and daunting illness. Our task was to serve as their guides for the journey.

When Saar began his cancer treatment, we called on his friends and colleagues in the cancer community, including Gabe Hortobagyi, MD, chair of breast oncology at the M. D. Anderson Cancer Center, and Lydia Mouzaka, MD, an international leader in cancer research.

Our own search for guides led us to national and local experts in multiple myeloma and leukemia. They were, as we discovered, the closest Saar would come to specialists in his type of cancer, which had no cutting-edge treatments or experts of its own.

Once we had gathered four opinions, we set about making decisions. We based our choices on the expertise of various doctors and their willingness to work with us as partners. Dan Stepan, MD, the treating medical oncologist, agreed that Saar should be part of the decision-making process. Dan and Brian Durie, MD, an international expert and research medical oncologist, would serve as local consultants. Ray Alexanian, MD, another international expert and research med-

James's Discovery

James, a 55-year-old sports public relations executive, had just begun chemotherapy for lymphoma—going for a remission—when he started having fainting spells. He didn't think they were a big deal, and he was afraid and embarrassed to tell his doctor about them.

Finally, after almost passing out and colliding with someone while behind the wheel of his car, James decided that he ought to open up. If he didn't like his doctor's response, he was prepared to argue about it or to seek a second opinion. He decided to take a chance.

"I feel really stupid admitting this," James said. "A big guy like me . . . I'm a jock. But I fainted the other day, Doc. Does it mean anything?"

"I'm glad you told me," his doctor replied. "You're on steroids. They often affect blood sugar, which can make you feel faint. Be sure you keep lollipops with you, especially chocolate ones. The sugar will get you through the light-headed times."

Relieved, James replied, "I'm so glad I mentioned something. I was going to tough it out. I was afraid you'd reduce my chemo dose and my chances for remission." His doctor answered, "Not this time."

Being strong and stoic was clearly an important value for James. But it prevented him from trusting his doctor. Had he silently toughed out other symptoms and signs, it could have been more dangerous. Hiding things such as side effects from medication or any pain or swelling (signaling a dangerous turn in the illness) can be risky.

Being frightened by a near disaster pushed James to overcome his embarrassment and learn how to handle his fainting problem. Moreover, it made his doctor realize that James was taking his treatment seriously and that he was observant and forthcoming about his symptoms.

ical oncologist, would step in as necessary to break ties on decisions and keep us abreast of the multitude of research projects at M.D. Anderson Cancer Center, his home base.

Saar had the final say in what he would and would not do. This allowed him to use the best of the best doctors and protocols. He also could deviate from the usual research-restricted protocol and customize it for himself—for his body and his needs. This is a unique arrangement for most oncologists and very unusual for most patients (but a growing idea, consistent with being proactive). Under the circumstances, it was the only one Saar would accept. It was agreeable to all.

Saar's first course of therapy was a steroid: a high dose of Decadron. It left him fatigued and in terrible pain, almost immobilized by muscle cramping. Stopping the drug was almost as painful; he said he understood how drug addicts must feel when going through withdrawal.

Over time, Saar and his doctors built in tapering-off periods that made subsequent rounds of steroids more tolerable. But the drugs still caused severe mood swings and sleeplessness. He became disoriented about the time of day. He was miserable; just being with him could be difficult.

As both his personal advocate and his cancer patient advocate, I advised Saar to see a pharmacologist, Robert Gerner, MD. Bob suggested adding doses of lithium at the beginning and end phases of the steroids. Normally prescribed as a mood stabilizer, lithium sometimes is used as a crossover drug for the side effects of cancer treatment. (Crossover drugs are those that have been developed for one disease and found—usually by accident—to be helpful in treating another.)

Saar started the lithium the day before he started the steroids, then stopped when he stopped the steroids. His mood swings subsided, and the muscle cramping all but disappeared. He still had some trouble sleeping, so he added a sleeping pill. This "cocktail" did the trick. He felt so much better. His quality of life bounced back.

A Remedy for Modern Medicine

Before the advent of modern technology, doctors relied on enduring, trusting relationships and common sense to reveal vital information about their patients. Often they knew families for generations, which meant they could overlay family history with verbal and nonverbal clues to interpret symptoms and make diagnoses. Perhaps most important, they took time to listen. They really knew their patients, who in turn received comprehensive, personalized care.

These days, doctors—especially the good ones—are overbooked and overworked. Most have good intentions; they really do want to help. But since they're so pressed for time, you must take advantage of every minute that they give you by planning ahead for your appointments. Be sure to take important papers such as your insurance cards and a list of your medications. Provide updates on any important developments since your last visit, especially changes in appetite, weight, energy level, sleep patterns, or bowel movements. Make notes of thoughts, observations, and questions that you'd like to discuss, and take them with you. Believe it or not, doctors tend to pay more attention to patients who use written notes. Besides, if you refer to these lists for talking points, you may feel less anxious about establishing a dialogue with your doctor.

While some advance planning can make for more productive appointments, the burden shouldn't be entirely on your shoulders. A true patient/doctor partnership requires willingness and initiative on the doctor's part as well. Unfortunately, even when patients work hard to hold up their end of the relationship, some doctors may not reciprocate. Many patients complain that their doctors patronize them, talk down to them, or rush them through their appointments. Some doctors are not capable of communicating well.

QUESTIONS TO ASK DOCTORS

GENERAL

1. What tests do I need at this point?

2. Are the tests painful? If so, is there anything I can do to reduce the level of discomfort?

3. How fast is my cancer growing?

4. How much time do I have before I need to start treatment?

5. How much is this going to cost? Does my insurance cover the treatments you are recommending?

SURGERY

1. Why am I having this procedure? What is its success rate?

2. Is there any other way to treat my cancer?

3. Are you certified by the American Board of Surgery?

4. How many procedures like the one you are suggesting have you done?

5. Are you experienced in operating on my kind of cancer?

6. Other than my cancer, am I healthy enough to tolerate the stress of the surgery and anesthesia?

7. Exactly what will you be doing—and removing—in this procedure and why?

8. How long will the surgery take?

9. What can I expect after the procedure? Will I be in a great deal of pain? Will I have drains or catheters?

10. How will my body be affected by the surgery?

11. How long will I need to recover? Will any of the side effects be permanent?

12. How long will I be in the hospital after the surgery?

13. What are the potential risks and side effects of this procedure?

14. What are the chances of death or disability?

15. What will happen if I choose not to have the surgery?

16. What are the chances that the procedure will cure my cancer?

(continued)

QUESTIONS TO ASK DOCTORS

RADIATION

1. What is the purpose of radiation treatment for my cancer? For example, will it obliterate the tumor or shrink it? Will it prevent or curtail the spread of cancer?

2. *If radiation is to follow surgery or chemotherapy:* Is this treatment intended to destroy any remaining cancer cells? Could radiation be used alone instead of with surgery/chemotherapy?

3. *If the cancer has recurred or spread to other organs:* Why is radiation being suggested? Will it destroy the spreading cancer cells? Will it control further spread? Is it being recommended primarily to relieve symptoms such as pain or bleeding?

4. What are the chances radiation will work?

5. What are the long- and short-term risks of this radiation protocol to any area of the body?

6. Are there other ways to achieve the same goals?

7. How much will radiation treatment cost? Will it be covered by my insurance?

CHEMOTHERAPY

1. What is the purpose of chemotherapy for my cancer? Is it expected to kill all the malignant cells in my body so that my disease will be cured or brought to remission? Or is it intended to relieve the symptoms I'm experiencing, without necessarily stopping the disease?

2. *If the chemotherapy is to follow surgery and/or radiation:* Is this treatment designed to destroy stray cancer cells that may have been missed by the initial treatment? What are the chances that my cancer will recur if I don't have chemotherapy? Will it improve my chances of cure?

3. What are the potential risks and side effects of the drugs I'll be taking? How do they compare with other treatments or with not receiving any treatment at all?

4. How will I be taking my medication? How often? For how long? Will I be given the drugs in the hospital or at my doctor's office?

5. Are there ways to prepare for the treatment? Are there ways to reduce the side effects?

6. Will my diet be restricted? My activity? Will I need to take a leave of absence from work or curtail my hours? Will I feel like exercising or pursuing hobbies?

7. How much will chemotherapy cost? Will it be covered by my insurance?

A study published in the *Journal of Family Practice* identified dissatisfaction with personal interaction, poor communication of information, and lack of trust in primary care physicians as the major reasons that about 20 percent of Massachusetts state employees switched health plans between 1996 and 1999. In a similar survey conducted by the Bayer Institute, West Haven, Connecticut, 25 percent of adults said that they had changed physicians solely because of communication issues. Most of these people never told their doctors why they left. Perhaps a report on another survey, published in the January 1999 issue of the *Journal of the American Medical Association*, got to the root of the problem. The report stated that physicians listen to patients' concerns for about 23 seconds, on average, before interrupting with questions.

You probably can't change your doctor's communication style. But you can take it into account when choosing a doctor in the first place. You also should tell your doctor when he or she doesn't seem to be listening or explaining clearly. If you feel that you're up against a wall of resistance, remember that you do have the option of switching to someone else.

PCMS Tool #3.7: Ask the Right Questions

How can you be sure to make the most of your face time with your doctor? Use these pointers to help guide your conversation.

- Be thorough.

- Be honest. It's tempting to say what you think your doctor wants to hear—that you're smoking less or drinking less, for example. But your doctor will be better able to help if you tell the truth.

- Identify what's working for you and what's not.

- Stick to your point. For example, give a brief description of your symptoms—when they started, how often they occur, whether they're getting worse or better. Think of precise adjectives to describe your pain or discomfort, perhaps rating it on a scale of 1 to 10. Be able to locate it physically on your body.

- Especially if you're anxious, embarrassed, or shy, ask your personal advocate or a family member or friend to accompany you to each appointment. Explain what that person should do during your visit, such as taking notes by hand or with a tape recorder.

- If you don't know what a word means or what the initials on test results stand for, ask for an explanation. There are no stupid questions!

Perhaps you'd feel more comfortable working from a script, at least until you figure out your doctor's communication style. Feel free to pick and choose from the list beginning on page 87, and add your own questions as you wish.

DIVISION OF LABOR

TASK	WHO WILL DO IT		
	YOU	PERSONAL ADVOCATE	CPA
1. Get materials for your cancer notebook.			
2. Make copies of charts from previous steps.			
3. Get a portfolio and tote bag for x-rays.			
4. Photocopy and complete your medical history (PCMS Tool #3.1, page 59).			
5. Photocopy and complete your cancer profile (PCMS Tool #3.2, page 64).			
6. Photocopy and complete at least three treatment comparison charts (PCMS Tool #3.3, page 68).			
7. Identify several cutting-edge treatment protocols for your cancer.			
8. Investigate clinical trials online, using PCMS Tool #3.4 (page 72) for notes.			
9. Make a list of CAM therapies in which you might be interested.			
10. Talk to at least three cancer survivors about any questions you have.			
11. Identify candidates for your medical team, writing their contact information in PCMS Tool #3.5 (page 82).			
12. Build your medical team.			

S T E P   4

ANALYZE FINDINGS
AND MAKE DECISIONS

In the previous three steps, you initiated much of the legwork that's going to carry you through the remainder of the Personal Cancer Management System (PCMS). Let's recap what you've accomplished so far.

- You've chosen a personal advocate and perhaps a cancer patient advocate.

- You've invited family members, friends, and others to join your support team.

- You've started collecting research, online and elsewhere, about your cancer and the available treatments.

- You've made lists of clinical trials and complementary and alternative therapies that may be appropriate for you.

- You've consulted your primary care physician and the treating oncologist to whom your doctor recommended you.

- You've identified other specialists as candidates for your medical team.

- You feel you understand your diagnosis, and you have a good sense of your options.

Now you're ready to review and analyze this mass of information, narrow down your options, and make decisions about your treatment. This is when second—and perhaps third—opinions can come in handy. You also should weigh factors such as your ideals and values, particularly about quality of life.

But first, take a moment to celebrate your progress. You've done your homework, and you feel confident about being an active participant in your care. That sense of control can make all the difference in your outlook and your outcome.

NARROW YOUR TREATMENT OPTIONS

Beyond quality of life, a number of factors will help determine which course of treatment is best for you. They include:

- The type and stage of your particular cancer

- Your age, medical history, and general health status

- Your confidence in your treating oncologist and your trust in his or her advice

- Your willingness and ability to cope with the physical and psychological effects of treatment

Some cancers are so well known or predictable in their course that the scope of treatments is rather narrow. Other cancers are more complex, which means that a wider array of treatments is available. The complexity stems not only from how the disease presents itself but also from how medical science has evolved in recent years. Technology is developing at such a rapid pace that scientists can forge ahead with research much more quickly than ever before.

Breast cancer is a good example of this phenomenon. For a long time, it was thought to take just one or two different forms. Now it's known to be at least 25 different diseases, the majority of which have very unique, very precise, and very effective treatment protocols. Understanding cancer in a way that allows for more targeted treatment is the trend in most current cancer research. The sheer volume of ongoing clinical trials for cancer agents speaks for itself.

If your research has turned up a number of available treatment protocols and potential clinical trials for your particular cancer, as discussed in Step 3 (page 63), now is the time to comb through the information and choose the one or two protocols and trials that are of most interest to you. Be prepared to share them with your treating oncologist at your next appointment.

How can you be so bold as to tell your doctor what you want for treatment? As we've said many times before, your relationship with your doctor is a partnership. You aren't trying to practice medicine; you're having an important conversation about your health and your life. You are entitled to explore promising treatments and to ask questions about their pros and cons. If one of the options isn't appropriate for your cancer, your doctor can explain why. You owe it to yourself to at least put the information on the table, so you can move forward with the confidence and peace of mind that you really have made the best choice.

PCMS Tool #4.1: Analyze Your Treatment Options

The tool on page 94 is a modification of a worksheet in Step 3. In this expanded format, comparing information about the various treatments should be easier. Feel free to modify the format as you wish. Complete one form for each treatment regimen. Then pare down your options to the one or two that you most want to discuss with your treating oncologist. Make copies of the forms for your doctor as well.

PCMS Tool #4.2: Analyze Clinical Trials

Like the previous tool, this one is a reformatted version of a worksheet in Step 3. It allows you to compare clinical trials and conventional standardized treatments side by side. Simply transfer the information from one sheet to the other—and be sure to make copies for your doctor. Again, the idea is to narrow your options to the one or two clinical trials that are of most interest to you.

SEEK A SECOND OPINION

Even if you and your treating oncologist are in agreement about your course of treatment,

we strongly encourage you to obtain a second—and perhaps even a third—opinion. Most doctors and most insurance companies would do the same. Here's why.

- Doctors are human. They may misinterpret information or overlook important details. Often they're working with medical records that are inaccurate, misleading, or just plain illegible. They'd rather find out they made a mistake than undermine a patient's chances for recovery.

- Doctors can offer different interpretations of the same information. One might notice something that the other didn't recognize.

- Cancer is a disease that grows geometrically. If it isn't treated properly the first time, you may not get a second chance. Moreover, certain therapies can't be effectively administered twice.

- So much new information is coming out at such an amazing rate that doctors can't know everything out there at any given moment, even if they specialize in a particular cancer.

- If more than one treatment protocol is appropriate for your cancer, getting a second opinion can provide the necessary clarity to make a decision.

Some cancers—such as skin cancer and early-stage cervical cancer—have very clear treatment paths with very high success rates, in the 90 to 95 percent range. In those cases, a second opinion may seem unnecessary. Still, we suggest one, for several reasons.

93

(continued on page 96)

PCMS Tool #4.1

ANALYZING CONVENTIONAL TREATMENTS

TREATMENT NAME	
FREQUENCY	
BENEFITS	
RISKS	
SIDE EFFECTS	
SUCCESS RATE	
COST	
YOUR DECISION	
NOTES	

ANALYZING CLINICAL TRIALS

TREATMENT NAME	
FREQUENCY	
BENEFITS	
RISKS	
SIDE EFFECTS	
SUCCESS RATE	
COST	
YOUR DECISION	
NOTES	

- Patients, especially high-information types, feel more in control when they know that they've covered all their bases. Consulting multiple doctors helps them to have more confidence in their decisions.

- Reviewing a case history with a new physician is not merely a perfunctory ritual or service. Rather, patient and physician are confirming the accuracy of the findings in the records, as well as their agreement or disagreement with the data presented and conclusions drawn. The process is a safety net against misdiagnosis.

- Talking with another doctor can provide a fresh perspective on your cancer, even if the course of treatment remains the same. You may come away from the conversation with a clearer understanding of the disease, the treatment, or yourself. That will have a positive influence on the direction and outcome of your care.

Keep in mind that a second opinion is just that—an opinion. It doesn't mean tossing out the mass of information that you've accumulated to date. The purpose is to be thorough in evaluating and winnowing your options. Sometimes disparate opinions lead to an alternative that may not have been apparent otherwise.

PCMS Tool #4.3: Use RECE to Get a Second Opinion

Chances are that if you're feeling any reticence about soliciting a second opinion, it's coming from one of those internal obstacles or resistors that we talked about in Step 1 (page 12). Sometimes we're afraid to challenge our doctors, who seem to have the same irrefutable authority over us as adults that our parents had when we were children.

Once I was visiting a friend when her teenage son's friend, Scott, stopped by the house. As the hour drew late, my friend suggested that Scott call his parents and ask for an extended curfew. Scott looked at his watch and panicked. "I have to get home," he said. "My father will kill me." I saw him and his father on the street a few weeks later. His father was 5 feet 9 inches tall, about 160 pounds, very gentle and soft-spoken. Scott was 6 feet and built like a linebacker.

Scott's instant reaction isn't that far afield from our own when we're facing the prospect of talking with our doctors as peers rather than superiors. But the best doctors don't claim to know everything. Rather, they're smart enough to tap their resources to get the information they need. More than likely, your doctor will welcome a second opinion. If that's not the case, it may be your cue to shop around for someone else.

You may recognize the exercise on page 98—RECE, for recognize, empathize and engage, collaborate, empower—from Step 2. Here we show how you might broach the topic of a second opinion with your physician.

Where to Find a Second Opinion

The same search strategies that brought together your medical team can help identify

Kathy's Conflicting Opinions

Kathy is a successful businesswoman in her early forties. She is married to Len, a lawyer who lost both his first wife and an infant son to cancer. For years, Kathy had been going to the Breast Center for her annual exams. She always left with good news. Then during one appointment, Saar told her that he had found a cancerous lump in her breast.

Because the lump was small and discovered at an early stage, Saar felt there was a good chance for a cure. He encouraged Kathy to be hopeful and, in discussing next steps, referred her to a breast surgeon for a biopsy. The surgeon found minimal lymph node involvement, meaning that the disease had spread beyond the original site into one node, requiring more than surgery. Saar referred Kathy to a medical oncologist for chemotherapy.

While Kathy liked the surgeon, she did not appreciate the oncologist's reaction to her desire to add complementary and alternative therapies to the chemotherapy protocol that he was recommending. He more or less pooh-poohed disciplines such as chiropractic and herbal therapy. Kathy, on the other hand, was known for her enthusiasm for holistic medicine.

Because of the oncologist's attitude, Kathy wanted to get another doctor's input. But her husband wanted her to forgo the second opinion and begin treatment as quickly as possible. So did her surgeon. The chorus of well-meaning advisors overwhelmed her and awakened the resistors that had been rooted in her since childhood. She became convinced that everyone around her knew more than she and that she was behaving ridiculously—even recklessly—by delaying treatment.

Saar knew that from this "stuck" place, Kathy would be unable to push aside her resistors. He supported her more proactive adult self.

Eventually, Len came around. Kathy then felt able to confront her oncologist and ask for a second opinion—and she was amazed that she had been so frozen when her life was at stake.

After she went into remission, Kathy credited Saar with saving her life. She valued not only his medical expertise but also his willingness to act as her cancer patient advocate. She was grateful that he was able to step in and negotiate the impasse between her and Len. She was thankful that he helped her get "unstuck."

doctors who would provide useful second opinions. In fact, the members of your medical team may be able to provide some leads.

- Speak first to your treating oncologist, explaining your rationale for soliciting a second opinion and asking for a referral.

- Consult a national expert in your type of cancer. If you've not already found one, ask your treating oncologist to

USE RECE TO GET A SECOND OPINION

RECOGNIZE

FOCUS ON THE OTHER PERSON'S NEEDS AND MESSAGES RATHER THAN TRYING TO BE HEARD. ASK QUESTIONS RATHER THAN OFFERING OPINIONS.

I know you're really busy right now. When might we find time to discuss some important issues about my treatment?

EMPATHIZE AND ENGAGE

LISTEN MORE, TALK LESS. USE INTERACTIONS TO BUILD BRIDGES. MAKE A HUMAN CONNECTION BY EXTENDING YOURSELF TO SHOW INTEREST IN THE OTHER PERSON.

Going off to speak at meetings must play havoc with your schedule. Have you heard about any new developments in breast cancer treatment at these meetings?

COLLABORATE

BE SPECIFIC. EMPHASIZE THE POSITIVE AND USE THAT AS LEVERAGE FOR COMING TO RESOLUTION.

I'd love to hear your thoughts on the benefits and risks of Herceptin. Whether or not to take it is such a major decision, especially since I'm estrogen-receptor positive. Any insights you can provide would help inform my choice. Actually, I wonder if we might get a second opinion as well. It would be great if I could talk with someone who's comfortable with an integrative approach—who's open to combining complementary and alternative therapies with conventional medicine.

EMPOWER

RECOGNIZE THE OTHER PERSON'S IDEAS, SKILLS, AND ABILITY TO MOVE FORWARD.

You know about so many of the treatments that I researched. Perhaps you can help me understand them better. As we go about making appointments for specialists, shall we stay in touch by e-mail?

suggest someone. While bringing in a national expert for a second opinion has many benefits, you need to be aware of one potential disadvantage. If that doctor recommends an experimental protocol, the procedure most likely will come under the rigorous guidelines of a large grant and so can't be customized to your individual needs.

- Ask the rest of your medical team whom in the field of treating oncology or research oncology they most respect.

- Contact cancer survivor support groups as well as other cancer patients. Word of mouth counts for a lot.

- Go online and search for scientific articles by experts in your type of cancer. If the same names pop up at least 50 percent of the time, you've found the experts in the field.

- Visit your local library or bookstore for books on cancer by doctors and other medical professionals.

Ideally, you'll be able to arrange an in-person meeting with the physician who's providing your second opinion. If that isn't possible—if, for example, you're consulting a national expert who practices on the opposite coast— you might try a conference call between the doctor, your treating oncologist, and yourself. Keep in mind that some physicians won't provide second opinions without an in-office visit. Offer to pay a consulting fee. (Some insurance companies will pay for second opinions, so be sure to check your policy.)

To make the best use of your interview time, prepare a list of questions in advance. The questions in PCMS Tool #3.7 (page 87) are appropriate here as well.

The second opinion likely will include a recommendation of a treatment protocol— either the doctor's or someone else's, depending on whether that person is a researcher. You may want to enlist this person to join your medical team as a consultant for those occasions when another expert voice is necessary or a critical decision point is approaching. Either you or your personal advocate can extend the invitation when it seems appropriate.

Getting a Second Opinion Online

In our view, it's better to get a second opinion in person. But we realize that isn't always possible. These days, your doctor of choice may be just a mouse click away. A number of hospitals and medical centers offer second opinions online, for a fee.

If you go this route, be sure to do your research and choose a service that's affiliated with a reputable medical facility. To assist in your research, we've provided several links.

Armed Forces Institute of Pathology
www.afip.org
The AFIP offers second opinions on pathology reports. For the most accurate interpretation of the results, it helps if you can supply fresh-cut, unstained sections of your tumor specimen. If none is available, the existing slides will do.

Cleveland Clinic
www.eclevelandclinic.org/eCCHome.jsp

Sonia sat opposite Dr. Gerber, her oncologist. She was barely able to focus on what he was saying. She couldn't get beyond the R word: *recurrence*. The breast cancer that she had so handily defeated 3 years earlier and never expected to see again was back.

Sonia heard her doctor say something about aggressive chemotherapy to "slay the dragon." She wasn't thrilled about the idea but thought, "I have to do something. Why not? Let's take out the big guns and do the job right!"

As a proactive patient, Sonia made sure to get copies of all her test results, so she could monitor them with her doctor. She even made weekly appointments with him, to keep close tabs on her progress.

As treatment proceeded, Sonia's disease responded and her tumor markers looked good. Then suddenly, the marker numbers were sliding in the wrong direction. Sonia

pointed it out to Dr. Gerber, who had missed several of their appointments for travel and other reasons. When they finally met, he seemed unworried.

The time between appointments was getting too long for Sonia's comfort. She complained about Dr. Gerber's apparent nonchalance to anyone who would listen. But she couldn't bring herself to get a second opinion. She was afraid that she'd insult Dr. Gerber by consulting another physician behind his back.

As Sonia's alarm at her rising markers grew, her friends and I put together a list of doctors to call. She tried to ask for Dr. Gerber's approval, but the words wouldn't come out. She was embarrassed and angry with herself.

Finally, Sonia confronted Dr. Gerber. He apologized for not staying on top of her test results. But she could not go the next

---

Cleveland Clinic experts will review your medical records and diagnostic tests and render an opinion, including treatment options.

Sidney Kimmel Comprehensive Cancer Center at Johns Hopkins
www.hopkinskimmelcancercenter.org
The center offers programs in clinical and laboratory research, cancer education, community outreach, and cancer prevention and control. Second opinions—both basic and complex consultations—are available through the Web site.

M.D. Anderson Cancer Center
www.mdanderson.org
This Houston hospital, which has been treating cancer patients for 60 years, is said to be the largest of the national comprehensive cancer centers in the United States. It offers second opinions and outside consultation pathology services, for which the patient (or the patient's physician) must provide tissue samples.

Partners Online Specialty Consultations
www.econsults.partners.org
Through the Partners Web site, physicians

step and ask about a second opinion. She accepted his apology, and he put her on a high dose of a new chemotherapy protocol. By then, her tumor marker numbers were out of control.

In Sonia's case, whenever she attempted to discuss a second opinion with Dr. Gerber, this can-do, in-charge woman felt reduced to a frightened child. We seemed to have reached an impasse. So I asked her if I could call her grown children to lend their support. She reluctantly agreed.

Though Sonia's son and daughter lived on the East Coast, they flew to California to have a family meeting about their mother's situation. All of us sat in my office, discussing the behavior that was most unlike their mother. Sonia admitted that she had lost control of the situation to anxiety and fear—that if she were to challenge her doctor's authority, he would abandon her.

That's why she fell mute whenever she tried to broach the subject of a second opinion. She felt defeated.

Sonia's son suggested telling Dr. Gerber that they wanted to consult a national expert in the city in which he lived (which he had wanted her to do anyway). Both of her children offered to go with her to do the asking and to write a script for her just in case Dr. Gerber asked if this was her decision. The family asked if I would provide a referral in the event that Sonia decided to stay local. She preferred not to ask her doctor for one. He had broken her trust.

Sonia called a few days later to tell me that the deed was done. She and her family scheduled an appointment with the expert oncologist. She thanked me for getting her "out of the rut" and asked me to continue helping her. Eventually, she went into remission.

and patients nationwide may arrange remote consultations to tap the expertise of the staffs at Massachusetts General Hospital, Brigham and Women's Hospital, and Dana Farber/Partners CancerCare.

ANALYZE YOUR FINDINGS

All of us know people who seem so confident and in control yet can't make decisions—even about something as simple as where to eat lunch. Throw a doozy like choosing a cancer treatment at them, and they'd be paralyzed.

Even if you're known for making up your mind with relative ease, you may struggle to do so when there's so much at stake. Yet you've got to do it because you know yourself better than anyone else does. Your personal advocate, or someone else on your support team, might be a terrific sounding board for your thoughts and feelings. Ultimately, though, you need to make the call.

"Who are you kidding?" you might say. "Whatever my doctor gives me, I'll take. What do I know?" Well, for one, you know a great deal about the quality of life you need and expect. Your task is to find a treatment that fits within those parameters. Here are several quality-of-life factors that you should consider.

Geography: You may be willing to travel to enroll in a clinical trial or to consult a national expert on your type of cancer. That may change once you begin treatment. You need to think about whether leaving behind family and friends—your support team—will work for you. If you'd rather stay close to home, that may rule out certain treatment options.

Inpatient versus outpatient care: For many cancers, some form of chemotherapy is the standard protocol. Physicians and hospitals vary in their practices for administering treatment. Some require inpatient hospitalization; others offer treatment on an outpatient basis. Unless the research guidelines attached to certain protocols dictate delivery methods, talk with your doctor about what's comfortable for you. You may want to inquire about a chemotherapy device that fits in a waist pack, so you can remain mobile while you're receiving treatment.

Cost: Health insurance policies vary greatly in what they will and will not cover. Some will reject claims for experimental protocols, while others pay travel expenses for consultations with national experts. A growing number of insurers are including certain complementary and alternative therapies in their policies. Be sure that you understand your benefits before you make any decisions.

That said, if you can't afford a treatment that appeals to you, move on to something less expensive. Don't suffer over it. Price doesn't guarantee quality. If you worry yourself into a state of despair because you're broke as well as sick, you'll get even sicker.

Side effects: All cancer treatment protocols cause some amount of discomfort, whether during administration or afterward. Find out what kind of side effects you can expect with each treatment, as they should be factors in your decision.

PCMS Tool #4.4: Decide What's Important to You

To help zero in on the personal and lifestyle factors that will shape your treatment choices, we've put together the values assessment tool on the opposite page. Simply read each statement and assign it a value on a scale of 1 to 10, with 1 to 3 being minimally important; 4 to 7, moderately important; and 8 to 10, very important. Once you've finished your scoring, scan down the two center columns. Here you'll see:

- Where your priorities are
- Where you are proactive
- Where you are reticent or shy
- Where some internal resistor is preventing you from taking control of your treatment and your life

De-Stress before Deciding

Making a major decision is tough. Doing it under the stress of a serious illness is even tougher. Stress can cloud concentration and impair memory; it can inhibit your ability to

VALUES ASSESSMENT

1. I prefer direction from doctors; I ask few questions.	1 2 3 4 5 | 6 7 8 9 10	I'm willing to ask hard questions of doctors.
2. I'm too anxious to take the time to investigate other opinions.	1 2 3 4 5 | 6 7 8 9 10	I want a second opinion, whatever the inconvenience.
3. I don't want to know details about disease and treatment.	1 2 3 4 5 | 6 7 8 9 10	I need to know all the details about disease and treatment.
4. I'm a low-information person; just tell me what's best for me and what I should do.	1 2 3 4 5 | 6 7 8 9 10	I'm a high-information person; I want to arrange for an integrated medicine approach and combine CAM with conventional treatment.
5 I want to be near a support team during treatment.	1 2 3 4 5 | 6 7 8 9 10	I'm willing to go to a national expert at a major cancer center for treatment.
6. I expect to be cured.	1 2 3 4 5 | 6 7 8 9 10	I'm willing to build on small victories to get the big win.
7. I need an authority relationship with doctors.	1 2 3 4 5 | 6 7 8 9 10	I want to build a patient-doctor partnership.
8. I need to stay with doctors and treatment that are insurance reimbursed.	1 2 3 4 5 | 6 7 8 9 10	I want the best treatment no matter what it costs.
9. The final decisions about treatment are up to my doctors.	1 2 3 4 5 | 6 7 8 9 10	The final decisions about treatment are mine.
10. Whatever it takes, I'm willing to try.	1 2 3 4 5 | 6 7 8 9 10	Treatment and side effects have to stay within my ideas about quality of life.

103

think logically and objectively. You need to clear your head before you set the course for your treatment. That means keeping stress in check, at least temporarily.

In stressful circumstances, most people instinctively seek out ways to relax and disconnect from the craziness around them. You probably know what centers you. If you've forgotten, or if you're so wound up that you haven't been heeding your innate desire for release, try these strategies for instant calm.

- Practice deep breathing (inhale as you expand your abdomen, exhale as you contract it).

- Engage in physical activity.

- Meditate.

- Listen to music.

- Go for a nature walk.

- Play with a pet.

- Spend time on a hobby such as fishing, gardening, or sewing.

- Watch a movie with your spouse or a friend.

PCMS Tool #4.5: Use Stop! Reflect! Clarify! to De-Stress

Do you remember the SRC exercise from Step 1? It's a great stress-reduction technique. Rather than distracting you from stress, it probes more deeply into its root cause. Armed with this information, you can be proactive about defusing stress before it gains a foothold. Use the blank worksheet on page

106; we also have provided a sample on the opposite page for your reference.

7 Steps to Effective Decision Making

With a clear and focused mind, you're ready to choose your course of treatment. To recap, here's the decision-making process from beginning to end. You can use this action plan to prepare for any major decision.

1. Identify the decision you must make. Ask yourself what most concerns you about it.

2. Gather information. Most decisions in the cancer process require some amount of preliminary research. The trick is to know what you need and where you can find it. Some will come from self-assessment, the rest from resources such as your medical team, support groups, the Internet, and your local library.

3. Identify alternatives. As you gather information, you may come across options that you weren't aware of.

4. Weigh the evidence. This begins the assessment process. What are the benefits and drawbacks of each option? Based on what you know about yourself and how much risk you are willing to assume, you can begin putting your options in order by priority.

5. Choose among the alternatives. Once you have weighed the evidence, you can reach a decision.

104

REDUCING STRESS Stop! Reflect! Clarify!

MY GOAL

_____

STOP! REFLECT ON THESE QUESTIONS

WHAT AM I DOING RIGHT NOW TO PREVENT MYSELF FROM GETTING WHAT I WANT?

Getting all tense to rush to decision.

WHAT AM I FEELING RIGHT NOW?

Overwhelmed and anxious.

HOW AM I BREATHING RIGHT NOW?

Too fast and shallow.

WHAT AM I THINKING RIGHT NOW?

I don't know what to do.

WHAT TRIGGERED THESE THOUGHTS AND FEELINGS?

Feeling that there's no time, no right decision.

CLARIFY FOR INSIGHT

WHAT IS THE REAL ISSUE?

I need to stop, buy time, and relax.

WHERE DO I STAND?

Stuck.

WHAT DO I WANT TO ACCOMPLISH RIGHT NOW?

Find a way to de-stress and chill out despite the decision to be made.

WHAT DO I WANT TO CHANGE?

Breathe slowly; clear my mind of fears; get unstuck.

TAKE ACTION

☐ Move toward my goal.

☐ Move away from my goal.

☐ Try a new angle to reach my goal.

☑ Change my focus. *From goal orientation to de-stress, relax, and let go.*

REDUCING STRESS Stop! Reflect! Clarify!

MY GOAL

_____

STOP! REFLECT ON THESE QUESTIONS

WHAT AM I DOING RIGHT NOW TO PREVENT MYSELF FROM GETTING WHAT I WANT?

_____

WHAT AM I FEELING RIGHT NOW?

_____

HOW AM I BREATHING RIGHT NOW?

_____

WHAT AM I THINKING RIGHT NOW?

_____

WHAT TRIGGERED THESE THOUGHTS AND FEELINGS?

_____

CLARIFY FOR INSIGHT

WHAT IS THE REAL ISSUE?

_____

WHERE DO I STAND?

_____

WHAT DO I WANT TO ACCOMPLISH RIGHT NOW?

_____

WHAT DO I WANT TO CHANGE?

_____

TAKE ACTION

☐ Move toward my goal. _____

☐ Move away from my goal. _____

☐ Try a new angle to reach my goal. _____

☐ Change my focus. _____

6. Take action. You've made a decision; now you must act on it.

7. Review the decision. This step will follow after you implement your decision. Have you made the right one? Are you seeing the results you expected?

Once you and your treating oncologist select a treatment protocol, there's little else to do but go for it. Feel secure in the fact that you've been proactive, done your homework, and made the best possible decision for you.

DIVISION OF LABOR

TASK	WHO WILL DO IT		
	YOU	PERSONAL ADVOCATE	CPA
1. Photocopy and complete at least one "Analyzing Conventional Treatments" worksheet (Tool #4.1, page 94). Add to your cancer notebook.			
2. Photocopy and complete at least one "Analyzing Clinical Trials" worksheet (Tool #4.2, page 95). Add to your cancer notebook.			
3. Get at least one second opinion—ideally, in person.			
4. Photocopy and complete the "Values Assessment" worksheet (Tool #4.4, page 103). Add it to your cancer notebook.			
5. Find ways to alleviate stress before you make any major decision.			

STEP 5

MANAGE SIDE EFFECTS

While treatment for cancer can bring hope for a cure, it also can bring—for varying lengths of time—side effects that range from embarrassing to painful. Often patients put off seeking relief, as if gritting their teeth and bearing the distress somehow improves their chances of recovery. You don't need to endure all that.

Some very effective prescription medications, as well as complementary and alternative therapies, can minimize or even eliminate debilitating side effects. By combining those measures that your treating oncologist and CAM practitioners agree are compatible—an approach known as integrative medicine—you build the emotional and physical strength that you need to fight the disease. The desire to reduce discomfort is not a sign of weakness. Rather, it is a sign of intelligence.

In Saar's case, as he listened to the members of his medical team explain what they thought would be best for him, he knew that he'd need to balance aggressive treatment for his rapidly moving cancer with his deep desire for a decent quality of life. He'd be taking a cocktail of powerful chemotherapy drugs, so we found out all that we could about them—

doing research, talking with survivors, and drawing on our own knowledge from our work with cancer patients. The list of possible side effects was long and not very pretty.

Saar placed a call to his good friend Gabe Hortobagyi, MD, chair of breast oncology at the M.D. Anderson Cancer Center in Houston. With Gabe's wise counsel, we put in place an action plan for managing the side effects, should they occur. They fell into five general categories: pain, fatigue, nausea, physical changes, and psychological/emotional issues. Let's look at each in turn.

PAIN

Pain serves an important purpose. It's a signal from the body that something isn't as it should be. For doctors, it's an important diagnostic tool.

In cancer, pain can result from the disease itself, as well as from treatments such as chemotherapy and radiation. As the cancer spreads or changes, so can the location, nature, and intensity of the pain. If not managed properly from the start, it will get worse. Over time, instinctive coping mechanisms such as stretching, deep breathing, and gentle exercise can't provide adequate relief on their own.

The latest advances in cancer pain management reflect the new understanding that the progression of pain follows an arc. By catching it early on, you have a better chance of getting it under control while it still is heading for its apex. Otherwise, it can set in motion a chain of events that triggers reactions throughout the body, as the graphic on the opposite page shows.

In the case of cancer pain, while some pa-

tients turn to complementary and alternative therapies (such as massage and acupuncture) for relief, for most the first-choice palliative measure is medication. Setting the right dosage and monitoring a patient's response are critical. Otherwise, it is possible to become overmedicated, which can have painful physical and psychological side effects of its own.

Far more commonly, though, cancer patients are undermedicated. In fact, in a survey conducted at M.D. Anderson, four out of every five oncologists conceded that cancer pain is poorly managed. Why is that? Some reasons include poor patient compliance because of medication side effects such as constipation and spaciness; poor doctor/patient communication; and patient confusion, especially in following directions to "take as needed." Doctors also cite managed care barriers, inadequate pain management training, and concerns about government scrutiny of overmedicating.

What every doctor and patient needs to realize is this: Untreated pain only gets worse. As mentioned above, the later in that arc we intervene, the worse the pain and its destructive effects will be, and the more medication we'll need to get it under control. It's like trying to sandbag a river after it has passed flood stage.

I remember my father being in terrible pain in the last 2 weeks of his life, after stopping his cancer treatment. I asked the nurse to give him pain medication. She said, "Do you realize he could become addicted?" As if addiction mattered by then.

Every step should be taken to contain and alleviate pain. Otherwise, it erodes not only your quality of life but also your ability to

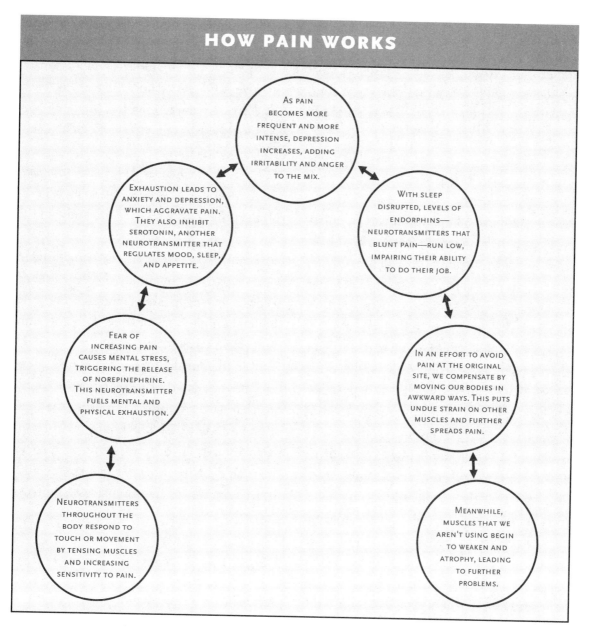

As pain becomes more frequent and more intense, depression increases, adding irritability and anger to the mix.

Exhaustion leads to anxiety and depression, which aggravate pain. They also inhibit serotonin, another neurotransmitter that regulates mood, sleep, and appetite.

With sleep disrupted, levels of endorphins—neurotransmitters that blunt pain—run low, impairing their ability to do their job.

Fear of increasing pain causes mental stress, triggering the release of norepinephrine. This neurotransmitter fuels mental and physical exhaustion.

In an effort to avoid pain at the original site, we compensate by moving our bodies in awkward ways. This puts undue strain on other muscles and further spreads pain.

Neurotransmitters throughout the body respond to touch or movement by tensing muscles and increasing sensitivity to pain.

Meanwhile, muscles that we aren't using begin to weaken and atrophy, leading to further problems.

heal. As we've seen, it will keep you awake at night, depriving you of much-needed sleep. It will cut your appetite when your body needs a highly nutritious meal. It will cause anxiety and irritability, which will make you hurt even more.

Over time, untreated pain will gain momentum. It will affect the nervous system, provoking anxiety, depression, and other psychological/emotional responses. It could be demoralizing spiritually. It also will trigger the release of hormones that adversely affect the immune system, such as cortisol. Maintaining healthy immune function is critical to beating cancer. One study found that people given morphine, a powerful painkiller, healed more quickly after surgery. In another study, involving rats with tumors, those treated with morphine lived longer than those not treated with the drug.

In short, pain sets in motion a vicious downward spiral. But it's one that can—and should—be broken. Relatively speaking, pain is a distraction. You don't want to waste your time and energy on it when so much more is at stake.

Getting Relief

As our understanding of cancer pain has evolved, so have the treatments for it. These days, doctors distinguish between pain *control*, which aims to stop pain at a specific site, and pain *management*, which involves getting ahead of pain as it moves across its arc.

Let's say you have a headache, and you place a cold compress on your forehead for relief. That's pain control. If you're prone to headaches, you might take steps to find out what's behind them, then address the underlying cause. Your doctor may order diagnostic tests to rule out anything serious. Once you get the all-clear, you might try therapeutic massage to ease muscle tension or chiropractic to rebalance your body. Or you might turn to over-the-counter or prescription pain relievers. The objective is to get ahead of the pain, so you can reduce the likelihood of future headaches. That's pain management.

In effective pain management, the farther ahead of the pain you stay, the more comfortable you'll be and the less medication you'll require. A good treating oncologist will anticipate your pain and recommend strategies for alleviating it. You can help by being as specific as possible when explaining how you feel.

For example, rate your pain on a scale from 1 to 10. Describe it with adjectives and/or similes, no matter how melodramatic you may think you sound: "It feels like very tiny, sharply pointed pins and needles." Notice whether it has any triggers, such as certain foods or activities.

Try to identify the center of your pain. This may not be as simple as it sounds. Neurotransmitters exist all over the body, so the pain you feel in one part of your body may be an "echo" of, or a response to, something in another part of your body. For example, a headache can originate from tension or poor alignment in the neck or back. This phenomenon is known as referred pain.

Should your doctor prescribe pain medication, you may try several before you find one that works well for you. From then on, don't hesitate to ask for it by name. In pain management, as in other aspects of cancer treatment, being proactive can spare you a lot of pain, not to mention stress and frustration.

Your Pain Management Team

According to a statement from the American College of Physicians, "Most cancer pain can be eliminated, and all cancer pain can be controlled." We happen to agree. In fact, pain management has become so integral to cancer treatment that patients are encouraged to consult pain management specialists soon after diagnosis. By collaborating with these practitioners early on, patients can put a pain management plan in place before it becomes necessary.

That cancer pain management has become so specialized is a testament to its recognition as a major factor in treatment outcomes, as well as quality of life. The advances in this field are occurring so quickly that treating oncologists can't always keep up. That's why they defer to colleagues who study and practice pain medicine. The health care industry has responded in kind, offering patients even more resources for pain relief. Among them:

Hospital-based pain management centers: Many hospitals, especially those that specialize in cancer treatment, have entire departments that focus solely on helping patients reduce their pain. If your hospital has such a department, ask your treating oncologist or any hospital staff member to meet with one of its representatives.

Private pain management clinics: Private clinics tend to offer a larger range of services than hospitals do. They also can feel more personal, with a less institutionalized environment and more customized care. You get to choose your own practitioners from a larger pool. Ask your treating oncologist to recommend a clinic in your area. Short of that, check online or in the Yellow Pages.

Your own pain management team: Much as you handpicked a medical team to meet your unique needs and preferences, you can assemble your own pain management team. Your treating oncologist—or your cancer patient advocate, if you have one—may be able to offer referrals. If you go this route, it's critical that every person on your team knows about every pain re-

lief measure that you're using.

In any of these scenarios, your pain management team likely would consist of some combination of the following health care professionals.

- Psychologist
- Psychiatrist
- Pharmacologist
- Physical therapist
- Occupational therapist
- Neurologist
- Anesthesiologist (for nerve blocks)

In addition, you might want to expand your team to include practitioners of various complementary and alternative therapies, such as:

- Acupuncturist
- Biofeedback therapist
- Chiropractor
- Energy healing practitioner
- Instructor of meditation or another relaxation technique

While each person on your pain management team should be knowledgeable, you also want someone you like and trust, says Edgar Ross, MD, medical director of the Brigham and Women's Hospital Pain Management Center in Boston. "This is a personal relationship that needs to be nurtured and developed," he observes. "It may not happen with the first visit. But the [practitioner] should be of the philosophy that whatever pain the patient reports is understood as his or her pain. There should be no further validation needed after that."

6 Steps to Manage Cancer Pain

Once your pain management team is in place, you can work together to create a plan that anticipates every level of pain and institutes measures for alleviating it. Remember, the key to effective pain management is early intervention—and that starts with you. You need to inform your team when you're hurting, where, and how much. This is why being able to talk with them comfortably and candidly is so important. (We've provided tools ahead that might help with this conversation.)

As you meet with your team members, you might want to share with them the following pain management model. It establishes a continuum of care to track with pain that ranges from mild to severe.

1. *Complementary and alternative therapies:* We recommend CAM therapies as a starting point because they are the least toxic. Your body will be exposed to plenty of toxins during cancer treatment; it doesn't need more. Also, with CAM therapies, you spare your body from the side effects of yet another medication. Acupuncture, chiropractic, hypnosis, massage, and meditation are among the options that have proven successful in controlling pain.

2. *Psychotropic drugs:* Mediated via neurotransmitters, these medications help manage emotional distresses like depression and anxiety, both of which aggravate pain. Since scientists have determined that neurotransmitters inhabit the entire body, not just the brain, psychotropics have become some of the most frequently prescribed drugs for pain management.

3. *Over-the-counter medications:* Among the most common OTC pain relievers are acetaminophen and nonsteroidal anti-inflammatory drugs (NSAIDs) such as aspirin and ibuprofen. They may be enough to alleviate mild pain.

4. *Low-dose opioids:* Seventy to 90 percent of cancer patients control moderate pain with oral opioids such as Darvon, Percodan, and Percocet. The long-term use of these medications has not been shown to worsen pain. If that should happen in individual cases, the patients may be advised to switch to an opioid other than the one they have been using.

5. *Slow- or fast-release opioids:* Perhaps the best known of the opioids is morphine, which is sold under several brand names. It's the most commonly prescribed medication for severe pain and is available in slow- or fast-release forms. Other slow-release opioids, which tend to have longer-lasting effects, include Fentanyl, Levorphanol, methadone, MS Contin, and Oramorph. In the fast-release category are codeine, hydromorphone, and oxycodone. When taken as prescribed, opioids—though quite potent—rarely lead to addiction.

6. *Invasive procedures:* For acute pain and some chronic pain, a nerve block can provide temporary relief. In this proce-

dure, the physician injects a local anesthetic into or around nerves or below the skin at the site of pain. The anesthetic interrupts the transmission of pain signals to the brain, providing relief for up to several hours. In some instances where drug therapy is ineffective, the pain pathways may be redirected or severed through surgery or controlled with implanted devices.

A Word about Addiction

Among patients, and even within the medical community, there is widespread fear that prescription pain relievers cause addiction. Perhaps it's fueled by the experiences of soldiers who were wounded in wartime and overmedicated with morphine, or by the emergence of a drug culture that has survived and thrived for the past 40 years. For the most part, the fear is unfounded.

That said, should addiction occur in the course of a serious illness, it may be the necessary price of getting through treatment. When that need is over, the physical withdrawal may result in temporary symptoms such as sweating or shaking. They're uncomfortable and unpleasant but short-lived. The key is to balance the risk of addiction (for cancer patients, less than 1 percent) and the effort to reverse it against the possibility of uncontrolled pain. The latter could mean discontinuing cancer treatment or lowering dosages, which could be life-threatening.

If you have a personal or family history of alcohol or substance abuse, talk with the appropriate members of your pain management team about it. Try to come to some rational balance between your fear of addiction or relapse and your need for pain relief.

PCMS Tools #5.1, #5.2, and #5.3: Overcome Barriers to Pain Management

If you're reluctant to seek pain management for any reason—fear of addiction or something else—you need to tackle your resistors. And the sooner, the better. You don't want to run the risk of developing severe pain with no plan in place to relieve it. By then, your doctor may not have any choice but to use the most potent measures. And even they may not do the job.

You probably recognize the tools beginning on page 116 from Step 1. They'll be helpful here as you go about identifying and confronting your resistors. We've included a sample of Tool #5.3 for your reference. For the others, please turn back to Step 1 as you need to.

Pain Management Resources

As we've discussed, pain management is a burgeoning field of study and practice. To learn more about the very latest innovations, you might want to visit the following Web sites:

- American Pain Foundation: www.painfoundation.org
- American Pain Society: www. ampainsoc.org/

(continued on page 120)

OVERCOMING BARRIERS TO PAIN MANAGEMENT

Identify Your Resistors

WHAT IS THE PROBLEM? _____

_____

A. ONE REASON IS . . .	B. ANOTHER REASON IS . . .
WHY	WHY
WHY	WHY
WHY	WHY

C. ANOTHER REASON IS . . .	D. ANOTHER REASON IS . . .
WHY	WHY
WHY	WHY
WHY	WHY

OVERCOMING PAIN MANAGEMENT

Take Control of Your Resistors

THE ANSWERS (WHYS) THAT REPEAT ACROSS SEVERAL RESPONSES ARE:

DO YOU SEE A PATTERN IN YOUR ANSWERS? DESCRIBE IT HERE.

DO YOU SEE RESISTORS IN THIS PATTERN? WHAT ARE THEY?

OLD BELIEF:

WHAT TRIGGERS ARE BEHIND THESE RESISTORS?

WHAT TO DO?

OVERCOMING BARRIERS TO PAIN MANAGEMENT

Stop! Reflect! Clarify!

MY GOAL

Overcome resistance to pain management.

STOP! REFLECT ON THESE QUESTIONS

WHAT AM I DOING RIGHT NOW TO PREVENT MYSELF FROM GETTING WHAT I WANT?

Being fearful and stoic.

WHAT AM I FEELING RIGHT NOW?

Anxious and stubborn.

HOW AM I BREATHING RIGHT NOW?

Okay.

WHAT AM I THINKING RIGHT NOW?

I don't believe in taking painkillers.

WHAT TRIGGERED THESE THOUGHTS AND FEELINGS?

They're a crutch.

CLARIFY FOR INSIGHT

WHAT IS THE REAL ISSUE?

I need effective pain management.

WHERE DO I STAND?

Stuck.

WHAT DO I WANT TO ACCOMPLISH RIGHT NOW?

Get relief from pain, which will increase my energy.

WHAT DO I WANT TO CHANGE?

Stop the tapes in my head; get unstuck.

TAKE ACTION

☑ Move toward my goal. *I choose to see the benefits in good pain management and get started on a program.*

☐ Move away from my goal.

☐ Try a new angle to reach my goal.

☐ Change my focus.

OVERCOMING BARRIERS TO PAIN MANAGEMENT

Stop! Reflect! Clarify!

MY GOAL

_____

STOP! REFLECT ON THESE QUESTIONS

WHAT AM I DOING RIGHT NOW TO PREVENT MYSELF FROM GETTING WHAT I WANT?

_____

WHAT AM I FEELING RIGHT NOW?

_____

HOW AM I BREATHING RIGHT NOW?

_____

WHAT AM I THINKING RIGHT NOW?

_____

WHAT TRIGGERED THESE THOUGHTS AND FEELINGS?

_____

CLARIFY FOR INSIGHT

WHAT IS THE REAL ISSUE?

_____

WHERE DO I STAND?

_____

WHAT DO I WANT TO ACCOMPLISH RIGHT NOW?

_____

WHAT DO I WANT TO CHANGE?

_____

TAKE ACTION

☐ Move toward my goal. _____

☐ Move away from my goal. _____

☐ Try a new angle to reach my goal. _____

☐ Change my focus._____

- Abramson Cancer Center of the University of Pennsylvania: www.oncolink.com (type the word "pain" in the search option on the navigation bar)

Another good resource is the International Association for the Study of Pain. You can check out their online journal, *Pain*, at http://www.iasp-pain.org/journal.html.

FATIGUE

Cancer treatments such as chemotherapy and radiation routinely cause fatigue as a side effect. It can range from mild tiredness to profound exhaustion—the kind that won't go away with any amount of sleep.

Unfortunately, doctors tend to do a poor job of preparing their cancer patients for just how intense fatigue can be. Only 10 percent of patients feel that they're receiving adequate treatment for fatigue.

The good news is, you can get relief. But you need to talk with your doctor—and, as with pain, the sooner the better. Your doctor may prescribe one of the following medications, all of which help alleviate the fatigue of cancer treatment.

- Aranesp
- Concerta
- Epogen
- Leustatin
- Procrit
- Provigil
- Ritalin

Not all of these medications work in the same way. Before your doctor writes a prescription,

we suggest asking about your options. Use these questions as a jumping-off point.

- Does this drug have any contraindications that would preclude me from taking it?
- Does this drug have side effects? What are they?
- Will my insurance pay for this drug? (Note that some pharmaceutical companies sponsor programs that offer these drugs at a reduced cost. For more information, see Resources, page 193.)
- How long before I notice a difference in my energy level?
- When will my fatigue go away completely?

You also might want to ask your doctor about complementary and alternative therapies that are known to alleviate fatigue. By adding these therapies to your treatment regimen, you may not need as much medication.

Energizing Self-Care Strategies

Beyond medication and CAM, the following nutritional and lifestyle measures can help alleviate fatigue.

- Eat balanced meals that contain a wide variety of foods. Emphasize whole grains, fruits, and vegetables, which are rich in energizing carbohydrates along with other essential nutrients. For protein, choose lean sources such as fish, skinless chicken, and fat-free and low-fat dairy products. Buy organic whenever possible, in order to

Shortly after our friend David learned that he had leukemia, his weight began to plummet. His body couldn't keep up with the speed at which it was losing its mass. His muscles weakened and went into spasms, causing what he described as "needles and cramps" all over his body. His appetite weakened, too, which only aggravated matters.

David spoke to his oncologist, who prescribed pain medication. But because his brother had died of an overdose, David was convinced that the drugs would become addictive. Instead of taking them in the proper dose, he bit off pieces of the pills. He believed that he could tough out the pain. And he did.

Unfortunately, David's weakened body wasn't prepared for the next onslaught of pain—this time during chemotherapy, when one of the protocols brought on a case of shingles as well as severe numbing in his hands and feet. David's weight dropped again, and the muscle cramps returned.

David held on stoically, believing that he was doing the right thing. After all, his tumor markers were improving. When his doctor again prescribed pain medication, David bit off pieces of the pills, just as before. He got little relief.

Elliott, a friend who was a cancer survivor, advised David to call Saar. Saar had been Elliot's cancer patient advocate, helping to guide him through his illness. As Elliott spoke, David's face turned cynical and guarded. Wisely, Elliott acknowledged that David was a private person. But Elliott had learned that private was not a good way to go. It would isolate David from the love and help of others. It also would prevent him from accessing important information and invaluable resources.

Shortly after, without telling anyone, David met with Saar. Together, they assembled a pain management team outside of the hospital group where David was receiving treatment. (Eventually, he agreed to let Saar contact his treating oncologist and explain what the two of them were doing.) His team included several practitioners of complementary and alternative medicine. He found that while chiropractic helped relieve all-over achiness, he needed acupuncture to help deal with more intense pain, as well as nausea. He saw a physical therapist for an occasional massage, which relaxed his tense muscles, and for help in starting a very mild exercise program.

David also consulted a pharmacologist, who recommended a combination of antidepressants and neuroleptics, psychiatric drugs that reduce neurologic pain. David learned that antidepressants are not just for depression. They target pain centers all over the body through neurotransmitter sites. With this knowledge, David was more comfortable taking the medication.

As he continued to work with his pain management team, David gained a sense of control over his treatment. As a result, his pain level decreased, while his treatment tolerance—and his morale—increased. Though he was not totally pain free, his capacity to manage his pain had greatly improved.

limit your exposure to toxins. Minimize salt, alcohol, and caffeinated beverages.

- Be careful to eat enough. Chemotherapy can cause anemia and alter your sense of taste. Both of these side effects can undermine your appetite. You need food to nourish your body, so you're strong enough to tolerate treatment.

- Engage in mild to moderate physical activity on a regular basis, such as a 10- to 30-minute walk around your neighborhood or the same amount of time on a treadmill. Your energy level will dictate how much you can do. Just try to do something every day.

122

- Get plenty of rest, including naps. Keep in mind that with fatigue resulting from cancer treatment, you probably won't wake up feeling refreshed and ready to go. Instead, think of rest as a bank account. You make deposits when you can, then withdraw when you need to. In this way, you might be able to avoid becoming completely depleted.

- Monitor how you feel throughout the day, taking note of when you are most tired. Let your body's natural energy rhythms help structure your routine.

- Tap your support team for help with chores, so you can conserve your energy for other tasks.

Help for a Good Night's Sleep

Many cancer patients report difficulty sleeping, which can aggravate fatigue. The cause of this insomnia can be physical or emotional. The following tips and techniques might help ensure the relaxing, restorative sleep that your body and mind need.

- Ask your doctor if any of your medications could be contributing to your sleep problems. With some drugs, such as steroids, you can adjust the time you take them so that they don't keep you awake at night.

- Make sure that your bedroom is as dark as possible.

- Set the thermostat to a comfortable temperature, according to your personal preferences. Some people prefer to run a fan while in bed.

- Choose soft bedding—sheets, blankets, and pillows—that feels good against your skin. Change linens frequently.

- Wear your most comfortable nightclothes, if you wear anything at all.

- Eat a light, high-carbohydrate snack at least 2 hours before bedtime. Carbohydrates help raise the level of tryptophan, a brain chemical that's a natural sleep aid. Tryptophan also triggers the release of serotonin, another brain chemical that helps alleviate depression. Healthy high-carb snacks include popcorn, toast or a bagel with jam, an apple, or a banana.

- Engage in gentle exercise such as stretching at least 2 hours before bedtime. Here's a sequence to try: Lie in bed or on the floor, face up, with your knees bent and your arms straight out. Drop both knees to the left while pulling both arms to the right, twisting your torso. Hold for 1 minute, then return to the starting position. Next, pull both knees toward your chest and grasp them with your hands. Hold for 1 minute. Now get on all fours and push back until you're sitting on your heels, with your arms stretched out in front of you. Hold for 1 minute. Repeat the entire sequence five times.

- Ask someone to give you a short, light back rub before turning in for the night.

- Avoid drinking anything too close to bedtime. Otherwise, you might awaken in the middle of the night to go to the bathroom. Be sure to relieve your bladder and bowels before going to bed.

- If necessary, ask your doctor about a prescription sleep aid. Non-benzodiazepine medications such as Ambien, Sonata, and Trazodone can help ensure a good night's sleep.

For More Information

The Oncology Nursing Society and the Alliance for Lung Cancer Advocacy, Support, and Education co-sponsor a Web site to help cancer patients deal with fatigue. In addition to providing information and advice, the site allows visitors to submit questions to trained oncology nurses and receive confidential, personal answers by e-mail. For more information, visit www.cancer symptoms.org.

NAUSEA

Nausea and vomiting result when certain chemotherapy drugs stimulate an area of the brain called the chemo-receptor trigger zone. Symptoms can occur within a few hours of treatment. Typically they last a short time, though on occasion they can persist from 12 hours up to 2 days. At such long durations, they can lead to dehydration and loss of appetite.

Because nausea and vomiting are such common side effects of chemotherapy, doctors group chemo drugs according to their potential for inducing intestinal distress: severe, moderate, low, and very low. At the "severe" end of the spectrum, producing side effects in 90 percent of cases, are cisplatin (Platinol), dacarbazine (DTIC-Dome), streptozocin (Zanosar), mechlorethamine (Mustargen), and high-dose cytarabine (Cytosar-U). At the "very low" end, producing side effects in less than 10 percent of cases, are busulfan (Myleran), thioguanine (Tabloid), vincristine (Oncovin), and hormonal agents.

For some cancer patients, the very thought of chemotherapy causes intestinal distress. This phenomenon is known as anticipatory nausea.

A Prescription for Relief

The medications to reduce chemotherapy-induced nausea are becoming more and more effective. With your doctor's guidance, you'll be able to identify the medication that works best for you. Among the most widely prescribed are:

- Prochlorperazine (Compazine), which interferes with the brain chemical dopamine

- Ondansetron (Zofran) and granisetron (Kytril), which block the brain chemical serotonin in the vomiting center of the brain

- Marinol, which fights nausea and stimulates appetite (it's derived from *Cannabis sativa*, the active ingredient in the marijuana plant)

- Aprepitant (Emend), a newer antiemetic

- The corticosteroids dexamethasone (Decadron) and methylprednisolone (Medrol), which sometimes are administered in conjunction with antiemetics but can be taken alone

- Over-the-counter antacids such as Mylanta and Tums, which are good for relieving mild cases of indigestion

- Mild tranquilizers, which short-circuit the anxiety that can worsen nausea

Depending on which medication you end up taking, your doctor could add it directly to the IV infusion when you're receiving your chemotherapy treatment. That way you won't need to take it orally, which you may not be able to stomach. Ask your treating oncologist about it.

More Solutions for Intestinal Distress

Your digestive tract is going to need some extra pampering through the course of your treatment. In combination with medication, the following strategies should help keep nausea and vomiting to a minimum.

- Eat slowly and chew thoroughly. Gulping down your food does not support smooth digestion.

- After treatment, stick with easy-to-digest bland foods such as skinless chicken, soft fruits, oatmeal, yogurt, crackers, and sherbet.

- Steer clear of fatty and fried foods, which tax the digestive tract. The same goes for spicy foods, gas-producing foods such as beans and tofu, acidic fruits, and sweets.

- Bypass foods with pungent aromas, since chemotherapy can heighten your sense of smell.

- Remain sitting up after eating, to help empty the stomach and dissipate gas.

- Sip liquids; you take in less air that way.

- Avoid strong-smelling tobacco smoke, perfumes and colognes, and cosmetics.

- Keep your home and workspace well

ventilated, as fresh air helps calm the stomach.

- Wear clothes that fit loosely around your neck and waist.

- If you're starting to feel sick, apply firm pressure to the inside of your wrist. This acupressure technique is an effective remedy for nausea and motion sickness.

PHYSICAL CHANGES

Potent treatments such as chemotherapy and radiation can save your life. In this context, the physical effects—weight loss, hair loss, and skin disorders, among others—may seem a modest price. Still, when they occur, they can be upsetting, even traumatizing.

Everyone has a certain perception of his or her own appearance, and certain feelings—positive or negative—go along with that perception. Collectively, they're known as body image. And body image is central to personal identity. So when someone's body image falters, it can have a profound impact on the person's self-confidence and self-worth.

By anticipating physical changes, you can take steps to prepare yourself—mentally and emotionally, as well as physically. In doing so, you increase your chances of coming out of treatment with your body image intact.

Weight Loss

More than half of all cancer patients lose at least some body weight during their illness.

About 15 percent of patients lose more than 10 percent of their weight. A number of factors contribute to this side effect, among them:

Stress. This plays out differently from one person to the next. Some of us eat more when we're under stress, while others can't stand even the thought of food.

Pain. When the brain is putting all of its energy into coping with pain, its responses to other stimuli—even pleasurable ones, like food—may diminish.

Treatment. All conventional cancer treatments can inhibit appetite in one way or another. For example, people who've undergone surgery generally don't feel like eating—even though their bodies need the extra nutrition to support the healing process. Radiation to the tongue and/or nasal area can bruise the palate, damaging taste buds. Chemotherapy often produces nausea that erodes appetite—though as we've seen, medications and self-care strategies can provide relief.

In cases where treatment impairs the ability to eat, a few sensible changes in food choices and eating habits can ensure that you get adequate nutrition. Our suggestions:

- For mouth inflammation or difficulty chewing or swallowing: Build your meals around soft, easy-to-swallow foods such as applesauce, bananas, cottage cheese, and milk shakes. In addition, your doctor may be able to prescribe anesthetic lozenges or sprays to temporarily numb your mouth.

- For dry mouth: Stick with liquids such

as soup, or liquefy solids in a blender. Very sweet or tart foods and beverages may stimulate saliva production.

- For altered taste perception: Sometimes cancer treatment causes certain foods to taste sour or bitter, while others lose their sweetness. Try altering flavors with extra herbs or sweeteners. Or just steer clear of the offending foods.

For more general help in addressing any weight issues, we suggest consulting a registered dietitian, who can develop an eating plan just for you, based on your nutritional needs and food preferences. In addition, certain supplements can support weight gain and/or help compensate for nutritional shortfalls.

To learn more about proper nutrition during cancer treatment, visit the National Cancer Institute Web site (www.cancer.gov) and click on "Coping with Cancer," then "Eating Hints for Cancer Patients."

Breast Loss

Women who've undergone mastectomy—complete removal of the breast—can choose from several reconstruction procedures. This is a situation where personal values and preferences count for as much as medical opinion when making a decision. We do suggest getting opinions from several breast surgeons and plastic surgeons, who can help explain the pros and cons of various techniques. Breast cancer survivors also can offer helpful insights. Among the procedures currently available:

Breast implants. An implant is a small pouch filled with saline or silicone that's surgically inserted into the chest to create a new breast. Often the procedure is performed on an outpatient basis. Because the implants are synthetic, they can develop leaks. Some may require replacement, depending how long a woman has them.

Breast flap reconstruction. This involves removing a flap of tissue from the abdomen or upper back to form a new breast. Because reconstruction uses a woman's own tissue, it can feel more natural than an implant. The procedure is more expensive, however, and it requires a longer recovery period.

Breast prosthesis. This is an artificial breast, made from material such as foam or silicone. It can be slipped into the pocket of a mastectomy bra, sewn into the lining of a regular bra, or attached directly to the chest with adhesive. The prosthesis weighs the same as the remaining breast, which eliminates any lopsidedness or back strain.

Sometimes during mastectomy, the surgeon must remove the adjoining lymph nodes in the armpit to prevent further spread (metastasis) of the cancer. With fewer nodes present, the lymph can't drain away properly. As a result, the tissue under the arm may swell, a painful and potentially disfiguring condition known as lymphedema.

If your doctor has recommended a mastectomy, be sure to ask about your risk of lymphedema, as well as possible treatments for it. Some support groups offer information on preventing this side effect, as well as measures for coping with it should it occur. Check with the groups in your area.

Hair Loss

Hair loss is a common side effect of some, but not all, chemotherapy drugs. Even then, it doesn't necessarily play out in the same way. Some people lose all of their hair, right down to their eyelashes; others experience only mild thinning. Still others shed no more than the occasional strand.

What's more, hair loss doesn't happen immediately. Your scalp may feel tight or tingly for a couple of weeks after beginning treatment. When your hair does fall out, it will go gradually at first, then in larger clumps.

If your doctor recommends chemotherapy, ask which drugs are in your regimen and whether hair loss is a side effect of any of them. Then you can plan ahead for it by adopting the following strategies.

- Before you begin treatment, get a short, stylish haircut. This will make the transition less dramatic and reduce the amount of hair that falls out.

- During treatment, handle your hair gently. Wash it with a mild shampoo and let it air dry. Avoid perms, colorings, and other chemical applications.

- Consider shaving your head. Sometimes people who have trouble coping with hair loss feel more in control when they do this.

- Once your hair has fallen out, decide whether to bare your bald head or cover it with a scarf or wig. Actually, if you're thinking about a wig, you might want to shop for one before beginning treatment, so you can match your existing hair color and style. Most cancer centers can recommend resources for stylish wigs. Seek pointers from cancer survivors, too.

Keep in mind that hair almost always grows back after chemotherapy. In fact, it could be thicker and curlier than before!

Voice Loss

Voice loss is a common side effect of treatment for head and neck cancers. In cases of partial or total laryngectomy, a speech therapist can help patients relearn how to speak. Also available are devices such as tubes that carry air from the hole in the trachea to the hole in the mouth, as well as amplifying objects that can be held up to the neck to increase sound.

For more information, contact your local chapter of the American Cancer Society. The ACS works closely with the International Association of Laryngectomees, an organization dedicated to helping laryngectomy patients improve their speech communication.

Skin Disorders

Chemotherapy and radiation can dry out your skin. With radiation, for example, the treated area may become red and raw. A prescription or over-the-counter cream or lotion can provide fast relief. Ask your doctor to recommend one.

Chemotherapy can leave the skin and nails paper-thin. When Saar went into remission, his fingernails tore and peeled painfully. I took him to my manicurist, who put on acrylic nails and replaced them every 2 weeks.

Opportunistic Diseases

Cold sores, skin rashes, thrush, shingles, muscle wasting—these are just some of the opportunistic diseases that can occur during or after cancer treatment. It's important to know that they are common and that help is available. But you need to be proactive. Tell your doctor about any unexplained symptoms, so you can get proper medication for them.

PSYCHOLOGICAL/EMOTIONAL ISSUES

Though cancer is a physical illness, it most certainly can take an emotional toll. The mind and the body work interactively. When one suffers, the other does as well.

Beyond outward emotional distress such as anxiety and depression, cancer patients routinely experience a more profound, perhaps subconscious sense of grief. Their illness is robbing them of their bodies; their familial, workplace, and social roles; and their very independence. The emotional pain of these losses can run deep.

It's important to recognize and address these emotions—whether through relaxation techniques, individual or group counseling, or even medication. Otherwise, all that negative emotional energy can undermine the physical healing process. In order for your body to get better, your mind must do its part.

I'm reminded of a parable about a monkey that roams free and steals ripened bananas from farmers. To stop the monkey's mischief, the farmers devise a clever trick. They hollow out a coconut, drill a hole just the size of the monkey's outstretched paw, and place a banana inside. Sure enough, the greedy monkey reaches inside the coconut to grab its prize. But unless it lets go of the banana, it won't be able to withdraw its hand. It is caught in a trap of its own making.

In much the same way, your body can become caught in the trap of your mind, if you don't take steps to mediate persistent emotional distress. By learning to let go of that distress, you'll be free to truly heal.

Take a Mind/Body Break

In Step 6 (page 131), we'll talk at length about the intricate connection between mind and body, along with the various complementary and alternative therapies that capitalize on this connection. The message here is that just as you can use your mind to overcome physical symptoms, you can use your body to overcome emotional distress.

One simple technique is mindfulness breathing, which makes a marvelous on-the-spot stress-reducer. This particular exercise is very similar to what you'd learn from someone who teaches relaxation techniques such as meditation or yoga.

- Close your eyes. Take a deep breath, then exhale slowly and deeply.

- Shift your breathing from your chest to

your abdomen. It should expand with each inhalation and contract with each exhalation. Continue taking slow, deep breaths from your abdomen.

- Become fully aware of your emotional distress—the anxiety, sadness, and fear. Don't try to shut off this pain. Instead, open up to it. At first, it may feel more intense; then it may come and go. It could transform into heat or a tingly feeling. It also could feel pleasurable, since pleasure and pain originate in areas of the brain that are quite close to each other.

- Imagine that you're breathing into and out of the pain, just as you're breathing into and out of your abdomen. With each inhalation, pay loving attention to the pain, rather than withdrawing from it. If this is difficult for you, recall a time when you felt whole, complete love. As you inhale, let that love penetrate the pain. Then exhale, using your imagination to break up the pain and release it.

- Continue for 5 to 10 minutes, or as long as you can. Repeat once or twice every day.

While practicing mindfulness breathing, try to refrain from creating expectations or evaluating the results. Otherwise, your muscles will tense up, and the emotional distress will return. Be an observer rather than a judge of the experience.

Incidentally, breathing exercises have benefits beyond helping to release emotional (and physical) pain. Healthy cells are aerobic, meaning that they require oxygen. Cancer is an anaerobic growth; as such, it hates well-oxygenated tissues. So by dosing your body with oxygen, deep breathing creates a less hospitable environment for cancer cells.

Constant Change

The French have a saying: *Plus ça change, plus c'est le même chose.* That is, "The more things change, the more they remain the same." Cancer will change your appearance. It will change your outlook. It will change your lifestyle. But it will not—cannot—change the essential you. That is, as long as you don't let it.

Ironically, the best way to prevent cancer from changing you is to accept the changes that it brings about, in the context of a larger process. That process is the whole of your life. You have been through many changes since childhood. These are just more. When you view them through such a long lens, they will not devastate you. They will not undermine your sense of self. In fact, they will reinforce your selfhood.

Consider these changes as an opportunity to pause and look back on your life. Recall an event that became a critical turning point, helping to shape your opinions, your values, your lifestyle. Recall another. And another. Now think about all the other aspects of you that have stayed the course even in the face of myriad other changes—a new home, a new job, beginnings and endings of relationships.

In Saar's case, he not only had to contend with the side effects of very aggressive treatment. He also had to adjust to the idea that in the very places where he once was the doctor and the expert, he now was a patient. Just weeks after his diagnosis, he wrote this in his diary:

There is a special camaraderie that forms between and among those of us sharing this experience. The first and foremost feeling is that we would rather not be sharing this experience. A pretty close second is fear. I feel a combination of shame and embarrassment for being here—for myself and for the other patients I encounter. I feel there is something wrong with me.

My way of dealing with this has been to turn the room I occupy during chemotherapy into my personal habitat. I pack a gym bag with the sweatpants and shirt that I don for sessions. I also pack:

- *My CD player and several of my favorite CDs, from classical to folk music, depending on my mood*
- *Several books on tape*
- *Two of the latest books I'm reading*
- *My laptop computer and a blank notebook and pen for writing*
- *My cell phone and phone book*
- *A blindfold and earplugs, in case I want to take a nap*

What I try to leave at home is a sour attitude—a sense of doom and gloom, of foreboding, of fear and loathing. In addition, following my own philosophy of inclusion, I make friends not only with the staff but also with other patients coming in for treatment. The whole idea is to turn it into a positive experience—a time to get things done and an opportunity to establish new relationships with people who will come to mean something to me.

DIVISION OF LABOR

TASK	WHO WILL DO IT		
	YOU	PERSONAL ADVOCATE	CPA
1. Assemble your pain management team.			
2. If necessary, address barriers to pain management by completing PCMS Tools #5.1, #5.2, and #5.3.			
3. Talk with your treating oncologist about other possible side effects, such as fatigue, nausea, and physical changes.			
4. Conduct your own research into side effects and potential treatments.			

STEP 6

SUPPORT BODY, MIND, AND SPIRIT

Surgery, chemotherapy, and radiation remain the first line of defense against cancer. They represent the standard, generally accepted approach to treatment—what most people know as conventional medicine.

At the other end of the spectrum is complementary and alternative medicine (CAM), which is gaining popularity as a component of a comprehensive cancer treatment plan. The word *complementary* refers to therapies that patients use along with conventional protocols. *Alternative* therapies, by comparison, are the instead-ofs—the ones that are substitutes for conventional medicine.

Although no CAM discipline has been shown to cure cancer, almost all that we'll discuss here—plus many others that you'll discover on your own—can reinforce and strengthen the healing process while you're receiving treatment. They're especially good at offsetting the side effects of conventional protocols, which—while offering the best hope for a positive outcome—can take a tremendous physical and psychological toll.

CAM and Immune Function

According to the Eastern healing principles from which many CAM therapies have emerged, CAM seeks to restore balance within and among body systems that have been disrupted by disease. Where conventional medicine targets specific tissues or organs for treatment, CAM considers the whole person—body, mind, and spirit.

A growing number of Western medical practitioners recognize the value of this holistic approach, particularly for conditions like cancer, which can have such far-reaching effects in patients. Through the lens of objective science, CAM appears to capitalize on the complex interplay between body and brain to strengthen the immune system, the primary defense mechanism against disease.

In the case of cancer, both the disease process and the treatment can suppress immune function. So can the stress, anxiety, and depression that routinely occur in cancer patients. These negative emotions originate in the limbic system of the brain, then travel the circuitry of the central nervous system via chemicals known as neurotransmitters or neuropeptides. For years, scientists believed that neurotransmitters existed only in the brain, but now it's known that neurotransmitter receptors occur throughout the body.

Coincidentally, the central nervous system is critical for regulating and maintaining balance within the immune system. If you think of the immune system as an army, then lymphocytes—that is, white blood cells—are the foot soldiers. Some migrate to the thymus gland and become T cells; others remain in the bone marrow and mature into B cells. The primary purpose of the T and B cells is to identify antigens, which are distorted or mutated cells, and to produce antibodies that destroy the antigens. Once the T and B cells complete their assignment, they are killed off as well, so the army doesn't get too large and out of control.

An excess of lymphocytes can cause trouble on their own. They can collect in the bone marrow, preventing the marrow from making enough red blood cells or platelets, which are vital for clotting. The lymphocytes also can wander into the bloodstream, crowding out red blood cells and causing anemia. They can collect in lymph tissues, leading to swelling.

If the immune system runs amok during cancer treatment, your doctor may need to alter your regimen—perhaps reducing the dosages of the chemotherapy drugs you're taking or the amount of radiation you receive. Treatment may even be suspended, at least temporarily. This can reduce the chances of a positive outcome.

Now more than ever, you need your immune system to perform at its best. Then it can do its part to fight your cancer, while you stay the course with your treatment. Certain CAM therapies can help not only by directly supporting immune response but also by alleviating the emotional distress that can depress immune function. What's more, CAM has proven useful for minimizing the side effects that often occur during treatment, which can ease the burden on your immune system while helping to sustain your physical, psychological, and spiritual resilience.

Even before he found out he had esophageal cancer, Frank had been a believer in complementary and alternative medicine. He decided that he would do everything he could to maintain the best possible quality of life through the course of treatment. This meant keeping his body, and especially his immune system, in good shape.

Frank understood that while CAM therapies would not cure his cancer, they would support his immune system. He also believed that CAM would give him the strength to tolerate chemotherapy at the necessary doses. He and Saar had talked about what might happen if he couldn't handle the chemo treatments: His chances of survival would diminish.

Saar, filling the role of cancer patient advocate, helped Frank to choose from the variety of CAM disciplines and practitioners available to him and to make the best use of them. Over time, his CAM team grew to more than twice the size of his medical team. It consisted of practitioners of both Eastern and Western healing disciplines— among them an acupuncturist, who helped drain the toxins left behind by chemotherapy; a chiropractor, who addressed the muscular and skeletal aches brought on by stress; and a nutritionist, who provided guidance on maintaining a healthy diet as well as nutritional support to counteract possible immune suppression.

Sometimes, when he was in a lot of pain, Frank would schedule an appointment with a massage therapist who made house calls.

He also maintained a rotating schedule of weekly appointments with a fitness trainer, a yoga instructor, and a physical therapist, depending on his ability to do more or less strenuous exercise.

As chemotherapy dragged on, Frank began to battle depression, fatigue, and sleep problems. He also became weak, which aggravated his pain. He made an appointment with Saar to find out if anything could be done. Saar provided a referral to a pharmacologist, who prescribed medications to address Frank's symptoms. Saar also recommended a psycho-oncologist, whom Frank saw on a regular basis.

Frank always had attended church regularly; he now found spiritual comfort in prayer and in talking to his minister. Sometimes his minister would visit him in the hospital during chemotherapy sessions. Frank also found peace through meditation, arranging to have a meditation instructor visit him from time to time.

Frank's value system played a major role in determining who would be on his CAM team. He liked that he could make appointments as he needed, with practitioners that he enjoyed and respected. He felt independent and productive as he stuck with his daily routine.

Whatever the outcome of his treatment, Frank found comfort simply in being proactive. He knew that he was doing everything he could to maintain his quality of life. And that knowledge gave him the upper hand in his fight against cancer.

Know Your CAM Options

CAM therapies run the gamut from the familiar (acupuncture, hypnosis, massage) to the unconventional (energy healing, macrobiotics, oxygen therapy). You may want to sample several of them, so you can select those that seem most appropriate to your needs, preferences, and comfort level. Be sure to discuss your options with your treating oncologist, who can then keep tabs on whether and how CAM interacts with the treatment regimen you're using. Your doctor may have experience with CAM and might be able to point you in the direction of particular therapies or practitioners.

To cover all the available CAM disciplines would require its own book. For our purposes here, we've chosen to highlight those with which we and/or our patients are familiar. To learn more about CAM and specific therapies, please visit the Web sites for the following centers.

- Memorial Sloan-Kettering Cancer Center: www.mskcc.org (under "Cancer Information," click "Cancer and Treatment," then "Integrative Medicine")
- National Center for Complementary and Alternative Medicine: www.nccam.nih.gov
- Richard and Hinda Rosenthal Center for Complementary and Alternative Medicine: www.rosenthal.hs.columbia.edu
- University of Texas M.D. Anderson Cancer Center: www.mdanderson.org (under "Diseases and Related Topics,"

click "Complementary/Integrative/ Altmed")

All of these centers support research to scientifically evaluate the efficacy and safety of various CAM therapies. Their Web sites offer information about clinical trials that are in search of volunteers.

Physical Support

The CAM therapies in this category may be among the best known. As you'll see, they appear to offer unique benefits for effective cancer management.

Exercise: Research has turned up so much evidence confirming the protective effects of exercise that the American Cancer Society now recommends regular physical activity as a cornerstone of cancer prevention. Even if you already have cancer, physical activity can facilitate the healing process in several ways. It neutralizes poisons and eliminates toxins from fatty tissues that have accumulated from the disease or treatment. It increases the oxygen supply throughout the body to repel cancer cells, which tend to prefer a low-oxygen environment. Vigorous exercise raises body temperature and increases production of pyrogen, a substance that enhances the function of white blood cells. As mentioned earlier, white blood cells are the immune system's first line of defense against mutated or abnormal cells.

Beyond its physical benefits, physical activity is good for your mental and emotional health. It not only triggers the release of feel-good brain chemicals known as endorphins, it also instills the sense of confidence and control that comes from the discipline of sustaining an exercise program.

Any physical activity—from walking to weight lifting—is good for you. If you're just starting a program, however, your best bet is to work with a fitness trainer or a physical therapist, or an instructor who specializes in the discipline you choose. This professional can design workouts just for you, based on your age, fitness level, and health status.

Acupuncture: Acupuncture adheres to the traditional Chinese medicine principle that energy, or chi, flows through the body along specific pathways called meridians. An acupuncturist inserts extremely fine needles along these meridians. Doing so can help revive life-sustaining energy and direct it to areas of the body that need it.

Acupuncture is of particular interest to cancer patients, as it appears to help relieve the nausea associated with chemotherapy as well as headaches, lower back pain, and other pain symptoms. It also may be effective in reducing anxiety.

For cancer patients who are receiving chemotherapy plus anticoagulant therapy, acupuncture may not be appropriate because of the risk of bleeding where the needles puncture the skin. As with all CAM therapies, be sure to consult your treating oncologist before trying acupuncture. He or she may be able to recommend an acupuncturist who has experience working with cancer patients.

Massage: Therapeutic massage—sometimes called bodywork or touch therapy—is great for alleviating the allover achiness that often accompanies cancer. It also stimulates blood flow, improves sleep, and counteracts anxiety and depression. Many cancer patients report that massage greatly reduces the side effects of chemotherapy, particularly on the day of treatment.

So many different schools and styles of massage exist that you should do your homework before scheduling a session. For instance, a deep-tissue massage such as Rolfing may be more strenuous than your body can tolerate at this time. Check to be sure that your massage therapist has appropriate training and certification and understands the unique needs of cancer patients.

Chiropractic: Chiropractic is of particular value to cancer patients who are experiencing lower back pain or other discomfort from muscle or bone problems. Practitioners of this discipline believe that illness arises from subluxations, or blockages along the nerve bundles inside the spinal cord. Chiropractic does not attempt to treat the illness; rather, it seeks to correct any spine-related cause of pain.

In chiropractic, as in all CAM disciplines, finding the right practitioner is critical. Your best resource is word of mouth. Seek out referrals from doctors, family and friends, and cancer survivors.

Nutritional counseling: By now you've heard the mantra: Eat at least five servings of fruits and vegetables every day, choose whole grains over refined, limit red meat and other fatty foods, and steer clear of alcohol. This is the nutritional foundation of cancer prevention.

You may throw up your hands and say, "What's the point? I tried to eat healthfully, but I got cancer anyway. It won't make a difference now. Bring on the steak and cheesecake!" In fact, you need proper nutrition now more than ever, to nourish your body and strengthen your immune system. By fortifying your natural defenses with key nutrients, you'll be better able to tolerate treatment and its side effects.

The American Cancer Society urges people living with cancer or at risk for the disease to obtain vitamins, minerals, and other nutrients from food sources rather than from supplements. We recommend consulting a registered dietitian (RD) for personalized guidance on an eating plan that matches your individual needs. Between you and your treating oncologist, you should be able to find a nutritionist who specializes in counseling cancer patients. Virtually every hospital has an RD on staff.

In some circumstances, nutritional supplements can be helpful, even necessary—although confirming their effectiveness in scientific studies has been difficult. At one point in his illness, despite trying a number of commercial protein shakes and supplements, Saar had lost 60 pounds. He was wasting away. His chiropractor recommended a "customized" protein shake that supplied vitamins, minerals, and other key nutrients, only without the added sugar. Once Saar started drinking the shakes, his weight stabilized.

Psychological and Emotional Support

Without question, cancer and its treatment can test the psychological and emotional resilience of patients. Yet just as negative thoughts and feelings can undermine immune function, a positive mind-set and outlook can foster the healing process. This is where certain CAM therapies can be helpful.

Individual therapy or counseling: Up to 40 percent of cancer patients report significant anxiety and depression. Of these, 9 in 10 link their distress to their diagnosis and treatment.

Talking with a therapist or counselor about the complex of emotional issues that arises with cancer can have tremendous therapeutic value. You're able to vent all of your anger, frustration, fear, and worry to a sympathetic ear—someone who can help sort through your feelings, provide a vocabulary for expressing them, and offer suggestions for managing them.

Some therapists and counselors work in partnership with psychiatrists and pharmacologists, who can prescribe medication to help manage more severe emotional distress. Of particular benefit to cancer patients are the psychotropic drugs. Originally designed to relieve anxiety and depression, among other psychological disorders, these drugs are now known to have broader applications. Specifically, they've proven effective in controlling pain and nausea, both common side effects of cancer and its treatment. They also help maintain healthy immune function. Pharmacologists, who conduct drug research in addition to consulting with patients, are especially familiar with these broader applications.

Your treating oncologist may be able to provide a referral to a therapist or counselor who has experience working with cancer patients. You also might want to check the Web sites of the following organizations, which offer online counseling and/or referrals.

- American Psychosocial Oncology Society: www.apos-society.org

- Cancer*Care:* www.cancercare.org

- Porrath Foundation for Cancer Patient Advocacy: www.porrathfoundation.org

Support groups: As we stressed in Step 1, an important aspect of outwitting cancer is being inclusive—that is, involving those closest to you in your treatment. Over time, your "inner circle" may expand to include a few new faces: the members of a cancer support group.

Back in 1989, David Spiegel, MD, professor of medicine and associate chair of the department of psychiatry and behavioral sciences at Stanford University, published a study on cancer patients who joined support groups. He found that participants survived nearly twice as long as nonparticipants—36.6 months, compared with 18.9 months. The support group members also reported 50 percent less pain.

The support group environment may not be appropriate for everyone. We urge you to attend at least a few meetings. Odds are, you'll gain a lot—and you'll discover how much you have to give.

Your local chapter of the American Cancer Society is a good resource for support groups in your area. You also may want to explore online groups, which may be a more comfortable and convenient arrangement for you. The following organizations can assist in your search.

- Cancer*Care:* www.cancercare.org

- International Psycho-Oncology Society: www.ipos-society.org

- The Wellness Community: www.thewellnesscommunity.org

Meditation: Meditation uses a combination of breath, thought, and imagery to relax the body. When Richard J. Davidson, PhD, professor of psychology and psychiatry at the University of Wisconsin at Madison, and his colleagues tracked 25 volunteers through an 8-week course in mindfulness meditation, they found distinct changes in brain electrical activity before, during, and after training. Mindfulness meditation emphasizes awareness of thoughts and sensations, unlike the more familiar transcendental meditation, in which practitioners focus their attention on one thing, such as a word or phrase.

Herbert Benson, MD, founder of the Mind/Body Medical Institute at Beth Israel–Deaconess Medical Center in Boston, has been studying meditation and other relaxation techniques for some 30 years. In his opinion, all forms of meditation offer measurable benefits for managing disease and promoting wellness. Indeed, the elements of meditation are similar from one "school" to the next and one instructor to the next. Here's a basic exercise for you to try.

1. Try to eliminate distractions. Turn off the phone. Ask someone to watch the kids.

2. Sit in a posture that you can hold comfortably.

3. Choose a word or simple image to which you can return if your mind wanders.

4. Close your eyes. Take four deep breaths, extending each inhalation and each exhalation for a slow count of 5.

5. Be aware of your breathing. Let it settle into its natural rhythm. Become a neutral observer of the "stillpoints," or pauses, between inhaling and exhaling.

6. Begin counting: 1 . . . 2 . . . 3 . . .

7. Continue for 10 to 20 minutes. You may open your eyes to check the time, if you wish.

8. When you finish, sit quietly for a minute or so—first with your eyes closed, then with your eyes open. Take a survey of your body. How do you feel? What can you see in the world that you could not see before? Wait for about 2 minutes before standing.

A number of books and audiotapes offer instruction in meditation. Among our favorite tapes is "Meditations for Enhancing Your Immune System," by Bernie S. Siegel, MD, a retired general/pediatric surgeon who has become a pioneer in humanizing medical education and medical care. Among the online resources are:

- The Chopra Center: www.chopra.com
- University of Massachusetts Center for Mindfulness: www.umassmed.edu/cfm/

Hypnosis: This therapy can help manage the symptoms of cancer, as well as the side effects of treatment. Exactly how hypnosis works is the subject of continued debate. Essentially, it involves deliberate, intense attention to a specific subject or sensation, effectively blocking out any physical or emotional distress.

SPIRITUAL SUPPORT

Everyone has their own definition of spirituality, their own religious ideology. Perhaps yours involves praying privately, attending a house of worship, communing with nature on walks in the woods, or simply believing in a higher power or a higher purpose in life.

Research from the National Institute of Mental Health has shown that strong religious beliefs loosen the grip of depression and improve the ability to cope with serious illness. According to other studies, participants in organized religion have lower blood pressure; a reduced incidence of heart disease and stroke; and lower rates of depression, anxiety, substance abuse, and suicide.

In addition, organized religion offers another opportunity for becoming inclusive. Religious congregations can provide a strong network of support, as well as a sense of belonging. Yours may even raise funds on your behalf.

Of course, it's perfectly natural to become angry at God or fate or the universe for a cancer diagnosis. Just as often, patients become angry with themselves. Spiritual practices, such as those mentioned here, should include forgiveness—especially self-forgiveness.

Prayer: Research examining the therapeutic power of prayer suggests that it can inhibit the growth of cancer cells, protect red blood cells, alter blood chemistry, and increase blood oxygenation. In some studies, even intercessory prayer—that is, prayer on behalf of someone who's ill—has helped expedite the healing process.

Pastoral counseling: Most religious institutions provide pastoral counseling for people in need. The counselors are members of the clergy, representing a particular belief system and using that system as the basis for spiritual guidance. Pastoral counseling also may include referrals to nonprofit organizations that provide services to those who are ill, such as Meals on Wheels.

From the Alternative Realm

As explained earlier, alternative therapies are those that are substitutes for conventional treatments. Indeed, many cancer patients turn to these regimens after conventional medicine has failed to provide a cure. Often alternative therapies promise a cure—though generally, they are unproven.

Among the available alternative therapies are the following:

- Antineoplaston therapy
- Hoxsey herbal treatment
- Immune augmentation therapy
- Metabolic therapy
- Laetrile
- Oxygen therapy
- Macrobiotic diet
- Shark cartilage
- Vitamin C therapy

We present this list not as an endorsement, but rather in the interest of illustrating the full scope of CAM options. Be sure to thoroughly research any alternative therapy that you may wish to try. Many online resources post information about these therapies. Among the best of these resources is www.mdanderson.org, the Web site for the M.D. Anderson Cancer Center. Through its Complementary/Integrative Medicine Education Resources (CIMER) page, it posts evidence-based reviews of published research involving a number of CAM therapies.

MAKE YOUR PICKS

The best choices from the CAM universe vary from one cancer patient to the next, based upon disease type and stage, treatment protocol, and side effects. Individual lifestyles and preferences need to be taken into account as well.

Ultimately, your choice of CAM therapies will evolve from conversations between you and your treating oncologist. Our hope is that you've chosen someone who's open to these alternatives. Still, don't hesitate to express a difference of opinion about a particular therapy. Be sure to poll others, too, including:

- Your personal advocate and your cancer patient advocate (if you have one)
- Your family and friends
- Cancer survivors
- Others who have knowledge of and experience with CAM therapies

Once you've narrowed your list of options, we suggest doing further investigation. While most CAM therapies are effective, some may be harmful under certain conditions. You can screen your choices by addressing the following questions, either through consultation with practitioners or through additional online research.

- What benefits can be expected from this therapy?

- What risks are associated with this therapy?

- Do the known benefits outweigh the risks?

- What side effects might occur with this therapy?

- Could the therapy interfere with conventional treatment?

- Is the therapy part of a clinical trial? If so, who is sponsoring the trial?

- Will this therapy be covered by my health insurance?

Appoint Your CAM Team

Once you've identified the CAM therapies that are the best matches for you, your next task is to find practitioners who can administer these therapies or provide training in them. Some major cancer centers have CAM or integrative medicine departments, with a variety of practitioners on staff. Generally, though, cancer patients must do their own legwork to put together a solid CAM team.

Naturally, you want people who have appropriate training and certifications. But you need to consider other factors as well—such as where they practice (some CAM disciplines are available only in major metropolitan areas), whether they're willing to collaborate with other members of your team, and how you will pay for their services if your insurance coverage won't.

The other side of this coin, of course, is that CAM is completely elective. You have the freedom to choose therapies that align with your personal beliefs and values, as well as your comfort level.

Back in Step 3 (page 76), we provided a list of CAM professions that you might explore. To recap, your CAM team could consist of any combination of the following:

- Acupuncturist

- Biofeedback trainer

- Chiropractor

- Clergy

- Cognitive rehabilitation therapist

- Dance and music therapist

- Energy healing therapist

- Herbalist

- Hypnotherapist

- Massage therapist

- Meditation instructor

- Nutritionist

- Psycho-oncologist

- Yoga instructor

PCMS Tool #6.1: Keep Track of Your CAM Team

As you screen candidates in each of your chosen CAM disciplines, you can apply many of the general guidelines that we recommended for assembling your medical team (see Step 3, page 79). Of the questions that you'll want to answer during your initial consultations, the following are most critical.

- Does this person have experience working with cancer patients?

- Is this person comfortable talking with your treating oncologist?

- Do you feel comfortable working with this person?

You can use the worksheet on page 142 to take notes, as well as to record each candidate's contact information. Even if you don't enlist a practitioner's services right away, you may want to follow up with that person later on. Feel free to make as many photocopies of this worksheet as you wish.

"I FAILED MEDITATION— OR DID I?"

All of the CAM therapies in this chapter are worth a test run. If one doesn't work for you, move on to another. Saar found that a number of disciplines he had recommended to patients were actually difficult or uncomfortable for him, as the following entry from his journal illustrates.

The fatigue—not the cancer—is what's depressing me these days. The other night I was wiped out by 10:00 p.m., yet I couldn't sleep either. I took a Remeron, wrote, read in bed . . . but another interrupted night.

The next morning, I talked with my psychologist about my exhaustion. He did not believe that my fatigue was the result of depression. He suggested that I meet with a Tibetan monk who is a psychologist involved in a project on meditation.

The monk, Lobsang Rapgay, is a study in contrast. He walks and speaks softly. The day I met him, he stood out from all the white coats and olive drab and khaki of the doctors and students at UCLA's Neuropsychiatric Institute. He was wearing a blue plaid shirt with a yellow flowered tie, blue pants, and red socks. "He is Westernized in education, but years of brilliantly colored robes seem to have influenced his standards in color coordination," I thought to myself.

Lobsang asked me about the fatigue, the sleep deprivation, and the frustration. He asked me to rate them on a scale of 1 to 10. I gave myself an 8 on fatigue, a 9-plus on sleep deprivation, and a "perfect" 10 on frustration. I explained that during extreme fatigue, my eyes feel as if they have sunk into my head, but my pulse does not fall. I can fight through the extreme fatigue for a short period of time, but it does catch up with me. If I stay up during the day, I still can't get to sleep or stay asleep through the night.

As for previous experiences similar to meditation, I explained that I had used hypnosis in the late 1970s. I even had performed surgery

CAM TEAM CONTACTS

	CONTACT INFO	ADDITIONAL NOTES
NAME: SPECIALTY:	Phone: Fax: Address: E-mail:	
NAME: SPECIALTY:	Phone: Fax: Address: E-mail:	
NAME: SPECIALTY:	Phone: Fax: Address: E-mail:	
NAME: SPECIALTY:	Phone: Fax: Address: E-mail:	
NAME: SPECIALTY:	Phone: Fax: Address: E-mail:	
NAME: SPECIALTY:	Phone: Fax: Address: E-mail:	
NAME: SPECIALTY:	Phone: Fax: Address: E-mail:	

after putting patients under hypnosis. I also had been able to do self-hypnosis, controlling my sleep, blood pressure, and pulse rate. When I tried it recently, though, I couldn't do it. I also had done biofeedback successfully; now I am unable to control my vital signs.

Lobsang asked me to visualize an object that was near and dear to me. I could not think of one but told him that I used to think of Sam, my lovable, graceful, black giant schnauzer. He asked me to try it now. I was able to picture Sam but not well enough to see good features. Nor could I imagine the dog in the room with me. Lobsang told me to try another object. I said that it was easier to focus on an object than a person, and he agreed.

I tried focusing on a yarmulke, a Jewish skullcap. I couldn't think why I picked it—perhaps because it was a symbol that I have known my entire life, even though I am not what you would call a practicing Jew. Of course, my wife the psychologist and my psychologist the psychologist would have a field day with the yarmulke image. They'd probably suggest that it is somehow related to unresolved feelings about my late father, who was a rabbi. He was, by the way, also named Sam. The connection may be worth pursuing. But I began to think that the answer was much less psychoanalytic.

I pictured black and white yarmulkes on a table. "Focus on one," Lobsang said. But try as I might, I could not get only one in focus. I did see similar shapes, such as a dome or semicircle.

He said that it was common to visualize similarly shaped objects.

*Encouraged to concentrate more, I closed my eyes tighter and furrowed my brow. "In visualization," Lobsang said, "if you try less hard and let it flow, it can be more productive and easier to see things." I remembered a book I had recently read—*King Con, *by Stephen Cannell. The con is pulled off by "holding on by letting go; increase by diminishing, multiply by dividing." Now I was relating Buddhist philosophy and visualization to a con game. What was my subconscious suggesting? That this new pathway was a con game? I knew I had to push my skepticism aside or this wasn't going to work. And I needed some sleep!*

At my next session with Lobsang, I noticed his color combinations had improved. If he wasn't getting to me, perhaps subliminally I was getting to him. He asked about my sleep pattern. I told him that I'd had 2 nights' sleep in a row, each consisting of a slightly interrupted 7 hours—a first for me in over a year. Though my treatment program was still stressful, I told him that my relaxation level was now 7 out of 10. The small victories were adding up.

As I heard myself talking, I realized that in challenging my skepticism—my resistors in sheep's clothing—I was embracing my meditations and getting better in the process. A bonus: Holding on by letting go was improving my golf game as well.

DIVISION OF LABOR

TASK	WHO WILL DO IT		
	YOU	PERSONAL ADVOCATE	CPA
1. Talk with your treating oncologist about various CAM therapies.			
2. Ask your personal advocate and your cancer patient advocate for their recommendations.			
3. Seek opinions from family members and friends.			
4. Poll cancer survivors about their experiences with CAM.			
5. Compile your own "best choices" list from the available CAM therapies.			
6. Interview candidates for your CAM team, using PCMS Tool #6.1 to record their contact information and any additional notes.			
7. Select your CAM team.			

S T E P   7

PLAN AHEAD

From the outset of treatment, your goal has been to send your cancer into remission. That can mean *complete* remission, with no detectable trace of cancer cells, or *partial* remission, with the tumor shrinking to less than half of its original size and the prospect of complete remission, should you choose to continue treatment.

Sometimes doctors will recommend a "maintenance program" of chemotherapy or radiation, in order to flush out any stray cancer cells. For the most part, though, remission signals the end of treatment and the beginning of recovery. That's something to celebrate!

Make a point of acknowledging what you've accomplished. Cancer treatment is no cakewalk, but you've survived it. Perhaps you can get away for a long weekend or throw a party for your family and friends. Do something to reward yourself, to say "welcome back" to life.

Then take a deep, relaxing breath . . . because you aren't quite home free. You are recovering, but not recovered. First, you must rebuild yourself—physically, emotionally, and spiritually. You must reconnect with the people and the world around you. You must tend to the roles, relationships, and interests that once shaped and defined you but now need nurturing after months of neglect. Of course, you must remain ever vigilant against the recurrence of cancer.

Saar entered remission 8 months after his diagnosis. We quickly realized that in the absence of a formal "road map" for the recovery process, we'd need to create one for ourselves. Saar turned to his CAM (complementary and alternative medicine) team, this time enlisting the services of a nutritionist, a fitness trainer, a cognitive trainer (who helps retrain the brain from the effects of chemotherapy), and a career counselor. Together, they would help set the course for his recovery and for his future.

LET GO OF THE "CANCER PATIENT" IDENTITY

While learning that you had cancer probably was terrifying, finding out that you *don't* have it can be just as unnerving. After all, you've made a career out of finding a cure for yourself. Now, in effect, you've been given a pink slip, phased out of the identity you had been forced to adopt.

More than likely, you'll say good-bye to people who sustained you through your treatment—like your treating oncologist, who addressed your endless questions with patience and understanding; the nurses at the treatment center who "adopted" you and took such good care of you; the librarian who helped figure out the guide to periodicals. Even your relationship with your personal advocate will diminish.

You may feel empty and lost, as though you lack purpose. You may wonder, "Who am

I now, if not a cancer patient?" This sense of mourning is completely normal. If you were to talk with a therapist, counselor, or another mental health professional (which isn't a bad idea), you would probably be encouraged to seek closure. You could show appreciation to the people who stood by you through your treatment by sending thank-you cards, flowers, or small gifts. You could write about them in your journal or collect their photographs into a journal. This is not morbid; rather, it honors all that you've been through. You've accomplished one helluva feat!

OVERCOME ANY UNCERTAINTY

Another aftereffect of remission is the seemingly nonstop swirl of what-ifs: "What if the treatment didn't get all of the cancer?" "What if it comes back?" "What if I need chemo again?" "What if it doesn't work this time?" "What if I can't have a normal life?" Living under a cloud of the unknown is its own source of stress.

Asking your doctor these questions may offer little in the way of reassurance, as he or she probably doesn't have the answers either. In the face of so much uncertainty, you may feel that your situation is beyond your control, which only elevates your stress level. That will hinder your recovery.

By taking steps to defuse your stress, you can see your situation from a fresh perspective—perhaps not eliminating the what-ifs, but at least giving you the upper hand. Here's what to do.

Identify other aspects of your life where you

don't have complete control. Back in Step 1, we discussed how some things about cancer are beyond anyone's control—and how acknowledging that can be empowering. The same rule applies posttreatment. It might help to remember the familiar credo of Alcoholics Anonymous: "God grant me the serenity to accept the things I cannot change, the courage to change the things I can, and the wisdom to know the difference."

Create or resume rituals. Whether it's a morning walk or afternoon tea with a good friend, the regularity of such activities will remind you that you *can* be certain about some things in life. Make an effort to seek out and engage in what you enjoy; it will alter your sense of time, lift your mood, and increase your energy.

Practice a relaxation technique. What matters most here is selecting a technique that you enjoy, so you'll use it when you need to. It could be stretching, meditating, deep breathing, or staring at a tank full of tropical fish for 15 minutes—whatever works to switch off your body's stress response.

Tap the healing power of laughter. Research confirms that laughter is a marvelous psychological defense against stress and its negative effects on the body. Laughter has numerous therapeutic benefits; it can:

- Lower blood pressure
- Boost energy
- Promote relaxation
- Alleviate depression
- Increase endorphins, the feel-good brain chemicals that enhance the sense of well-being

Opportunities to tickle your funny bone are everywhere around you. For example, you could try any of these activities.

- Pick up a funny book from the humor shelf of your local library or bookstore.
- Watch your favorite sitcoms, from contemporary shows to classic reruns.
- Rent a selection of laugh-till-you-cry comedy films.
- Spend time in the company of family and friends who make you laugh.

Head outdoors. Appreciate the timeless quality of nature. It will inspire you and help you understand your place in the grand scheme of things. That may seem humbling, but in fact, it will expand your sense of self when you realize that you are part of something much larger than any one individual.

Examine your beliefs about death and dying. It's impossible to experience a life-threatening disease like cancer without contemplating your own mortality. When you're ready, have a dialogue with yourself about these thoughts and feelings. If it's difficult for you, you might want to invite someone—a family member or close friend, someone from the clergy, or a mental health professional—to listen and guide you. In a paradoxical way, acknowledging your beliefs about death and dying chips away at your fear of recurrence. It also can help you shed your "cancer patient" identity and embrace a "survivor" identity.

Savor each moment. Life—your life—is a gift. By focusing on what you have, instead of what you have (or could have) lost, you come to appreciate the simple fact that *you still are here*. This will help you move beyond any uncertainty, any sense of victimization, that you may be experiencing.

BEGIN REBUILDING

Every person who goes through the cancer experience is profoundly changed by it. Now that you're in remission, it probably is a good time for some self-assessment—to look at where you've been, where you are currently, and where you want to go from here.

For this process to have a meaningful outcome, you need to identify what is most important to you—that is, your core values. These are deeply held personal convictions that some actions or goals are preferable to others. The strength of your core values versus other, more casual values gives them more weight. They coalesce into a value system that drives all of your decisions. When you stray from your value system, you feel a sense of failure, of disappointing yourself and others.

As you go about your self-assessment, you may notice a shift in your core values. Many cancer survivors do. Precancer, you might have placed a high priority on knowledge, drive, and discipline—all the hallmarks of a successful career. Now you're contemplating whether you want to return to work or instead invest your time and energy in community service. Of course, this raises a whole host of issues that you need to address. To what extent has your job driven your identity? Can you afford to leave full-time employment? What will happen with your health insurance? If you're unhappy, should

you consider switching careers instead of leaving the workplace? As you sort through your "new" core values, the answers to these questions will become clear.

Courage is another core value that you may need to rethink. As you now realize, it is not about being fearless; rather, it is about being afraid and moving forward anyway. You have shown tremendous courage by facing cancer and its treatment.

PCMS Tool #7.1: Know Thyself— A Values Survey

Through the series of worksheets beginning on the opposite page, you will consciously identify your core values, so you can apply them when charting your course for the future. As you'll see, the cancer experience will reshape your value system to better serve you in this new stage of your life.

Each of the seven exercises builds on the one preceding it. By completing the series, you should come away with a clearer picture of who you are now and what you want and need at this stage of your life.

Life Is Like a Jar of Rocks

As Saar contemplated what he was going to do with the rest of his life, he remembered a lesson that his father had passed on to him when he was a young man. Rabbi Porrath picked up a large, empty mayonnaise jar and filled it to the top with rocks about 2 inches in diameter. He asked Saar if the jar was full. Saar said that it was. Next his father picked up a box of pebbles and poured them into the

(continued on page 154)

148

Part I: Moral Values

Below is a list of qualities that define your moral core. Collectively, they form the yardstick by which you measure your self-image and self-worth. Please rank these qualities in order of importance to you, with 10 as most desirable and 1 as least.

RANK 1–10	MORAL VALUE	CHARACTERISTICS
	Affection	Caring, compassionate
	Honesty	Ethical, moral, truthful
	Service	Useful, helpful
	Tolerance	Accepting, open, patient
	Fairness	Just, unbiased, impartial
	Courtesy	Well-mannered, respectful, considerate
	Loyalty	Devoted, dedicated
	Forgiveness	Able to excuse and move on
	Obedient	Compliant, deferential
	Courage	Brave, intrepid—sometimes in the face of fear

Part II: Emotional Competencies

Emotional competencies are personality traits that motivate and drive behavior. They are part of your value system in that they influence your decision-making process. Please rank the following competencies in order of importance to you, with 9 as most preferable and 1 as least.

RANK 1–9	EMOTIONAL COMPETENCY	CHARACTERISTICS
	Knowledge	Having wisdom acquired through study and experience
	Drive	Goal-directed, industrious
	Accountability	Trustworthy, responsible, credible
	Creativity	Innovative, original
	Discipline	Self-controlled, focused, committed
	Autonomy	Self-directed, self-reliant
	Flexibility	Adaptable, able to change
	Reasonableness	Logical, rational, analytical
	Humor	Witty, funny

Part III: Personal Life Goals

What constitutes a satisfying, fulfilling personal life varies from one person to the next. To which of the following do you aspire? Please rank them in order of importance, with 12 as most valuable and 1 as least.

RANK 1–12	PERSONAL LIFE GOALS	CHARACTERISTICS
	Happiness	Satisfaction, joy, contentment
	Health	Soundness of body and mind
	Self-worth	High regard for self and others
	Wisdom	Insight, knowledge, understanding
	Achievement	Aspiration to succeed
	Wealth	Affluence, prosperity
	Pleasure	Entertainment, relaxation, fun
	Adventure	Excitement, risk-taking
	Fame	Desire to be recognized publicly for contributions
	Aesthetics	Appreciation and enjoyment of arts
	Spirituality	Feeling at one with God, religious beliefs
	Vitality	Energy, passion, verve

Part IV: Social Life Goals

Your social life goals shape your interactions with others. Please rank the following in order of importance to you, with 9 as most desirable and 1 as least.

RANK 1–9	SOCIAL LIFE GOALS	CHARACTERISTICS
	Family	Close, supportive relationships with loved ones
	Love	Relationships marked by intimacy, devotion, warmth
	Freedom	Relationships marked by independent thought, action, lifestyle
	Peace	Working toward lasting harmony in relationships
	Equality	Justice and fairness for all
	Fellowship	Close, supportive relationships with friends
	Social service	Concern, compassion for the welfare of others
	Community	Participation in social and/or community groups
	Power	Exercising authority, control, influence in relationships

Part V: Summary

Fill in your top three entries from each of the preceding worksheets. Collectively, these will serve as your compass as you make plans for life after treatment.

VALUES AND LIFE GOALS	TOP THREE IN EACH CATEGORY
Moral Values	1.
Moral Values	2.
Moral Values	3.
Emotional Competencies	1.
Emotional Competencies	2.
Emotional Competencies	3.
Personal Life Goals	1.
Personal Life Goals	2.
Personal Life Goals	3.
Social Life Goals	1.
Social Life Goals	2.
Social Life Goals	3.

PCMS Tool #7.1

Part VI: Interpreting Values and Goals

For each value or goal in the summary worksheet, craft a sentence that will guide you in applying this insight to yourself and your life.

Example (for drive, an emotional competency): I need to establish meaningful priorities to direct my goals going forward.

MORAL VALUES

1.

2.

3.

EMOTIONAL COMPETENCIES

1.

2.

3.

PERSONAL LIFE GOALS

1.

2.

3.

SOCIAL LIFE GOALS

1.

2.

3.

Part VII: Envision Your Goals

Close your eyes and relax with three repetitions of the mindfulness breathing exercise in Step 5 (page 128). Choose one of your values or goals. How do you see yourself implementing it in your life? Delve into the details of your vision. Then open your eyes and write down what you've just imagined. This exercise helps engage both the left and right sides of your brain in your values and goals, effectively "translating" them from information to action.

jar, shaking it lightly. The pebbles rolled into the open areas between the rocks. Again, Rabbi Porrath asked Saar if the jar was full. Saar agreed that yes, it was. Then his father picked up a box of sand and poured it into the jar. The sand filled up the rest of the space.

"I want you to recognize that the jar is your life," Rabbi Porrath explained. "The rocks are the important things—your partner, your children, your health, anything so vital to you that without it, you would be nearly destroyed. The pebbles are the other things in life that matter, but on a smaller scale—things like your job, house, or car. The sand is everything else, the small stuff.

"If you put the sand or the pebbles into the jar first, you have no room for the rocks. The same goes for life. If you spend all your time and energy on the small stuff, the material things, you have no room for the things that are most important."

As you look ahead to the rest of your life, remember that you always will have time to go to work, to clean the house, to fix the garbage disposal. Give top priority to what really matters. Go dancing with your partner. Play with your children or grandchildren. Get your medical checkups. These are the rocks. The rest is just pebbles and sand.

TAKE CARE OF YOURSELF

After cancer treatment, the best rehabilitation program is one that helps heal body, mind, and spirit. For this holistic approach, you may not need high-tech medical interventions. In our experience, simple lifestyle measures work best.

For the Body

As mentioned in Step 6, the American Cancer Society advocates regular physical activity as a cornerstone of cancer prevention. It can be just as beneficial to the posttreatment recovery process. Research has shown that a brisk 20-minute walk each day helps improve circulation and burn off calories (which can stimulate appetite if you've lost weight during treatment). Regular physical activity also alleviates stress, balances mood, and enhances energy and sleep.

You should ease into any exercise program, as your strength and endurance probably aren't what they were before treatment. Listen to your body; it will tell you just how much you can tolerate. If you're unsure of where to begin, consult a physical therapist or a fitness trainer with experience in cancer rehabilitation. He or she can help map out an exercise program that will return you to your pretreatment fitness level—and perhaps even improve on it.

Along with engaging in regular physical activity, adopting a healthy, balanced diet is critical to your recovery. Build your meals around fruits and vegetables, aiming for at least five—and ideally nine—servings a day. Fruits and vegetables are rich in antioxidant nutrients such as vitamins C and E and beta-carotene. Antioxidants help protect against free radicals, unstable molecules that damage the DNA in cells. Many experts believe that free radicals are responsible for the cellular mutations that lead to cancer.

Eating an abundance of fruits and vegetables also ensures that you're getting ample fiber, which has its own protective effects. Do try to limit your intake of fat and salt, which can compromise your health by contributing to other conditions such as heart disease and high blood pressure.

If you need guidance on proper food choices or are looking for inspiration with menus and recipes, consult a nutrition professional. Virtually all hospitals and cancer centers have registered dietitians (RDs) or certified nutrition specialists (CNSs) on staff. If not, they can provide a referral, as can your treating oncologist. An RD or CNS can tailor an eating plan to your specific nutritional needs and preferences.

Also important is getting an adequate amount of sleep each night. Your body uses this time to rejuvenate itself. While "adequate" sleep can vary from person to person, most experts recommend in the neighborhood of 8 hours.

Both cancer and its treatment can alter your sleep habits. It's helpful to turn in at about the same time each night. If you like to read or watch TV when you go to bed, choose books or shows that have a calming effect. Your body and mind need time to wind down in preparation for sleep. (For more tips on getting a good night's rest, see Step 5, page 122.)

For the Mind

As mentioned earlier, Saar's posttreatment CAM team included a cognitive trainer. Chemotherapy, radiation, and surgery can injure healthy brain tissue, leading to impaired cognitive function. Difficulty speaking, changes in personality and mood, poor concentration, loss of coordination—any of these could signal the need for some form of cognitive rehabilitation.

Ideally, you will have discussed the possibility of cognitive side effects with your treating oncologist before beginning treatment, so you already have a game plan in place for addressing cognitive symptoms. Besides, if you know what to expect, you won't be so alarmed when these changes occur.

Among the available cognitive rehabilitation techniques are biofeedback, guided imagery, energy healing, and music and art therapy. Your cognitive trainer also may recommend specific programs to retrain your brain. Many of these programs simply teach you to relax and focus, since just the stress of cancer can interfere with your cognitive ability. On your own, you can assemble jigsaw puzzles, complete crosswords, play computer solitaire—any activity that stimulates your cognitive function.

Now also is a good time to check in with a therapist, a counselor, or another mental health professional, even if you didn't feel the need to do so during the course of your treatment. The transition from "patient" to "survivor" can be an intensely emotional experience, as you mourn the loss of one identity and celebrate the arrival of another. Any change is stressful. Change of this magnitude can be *very* stressful.

Given your physical vulnerability at the moment, you have every reason to feel emotionally out of sorts about the impending transition. It's difficult even for people who consider themselves psychologically strong.

You shouldn't feel guilty, embarrassed, or apologetic about it.

If you decide that you could use emotional or psychological support at this time, and you don't have a mental health professional on your CAM team, you might want to ask your treating oncologist for a referral. Another option is to contact the American Psychosocial Oncology Society (APOS); its members are psychiatrists, psychologists, and clinical social workers who specialize in cancer care. To find a practitioner in your area, visit the APOS Web site: www.apos-society.org.

For the Spirit

Spiritual renewal doesn't mean that you take robes or enter a monastery, or even that you start going to church every Sunday. It may take a more subtle form: a clearer sense of your core values, a renewed joy in loving and being loved, a deeper appreciation for life. It's amazing how much the possibility of death and the realization of survival can teach about spirituality.

Prayer may have become part of your life while you were coming to terms with your own mortality. If so, don't abandon it now that you are through with treatment and onto recovery. Your prayers could turn from asking for health to expressing gratitude for it.

Another way to express gratitude is through mentoring, in which you share the knowledge you've gained through your cancer experience with others who are just beginning the process. Where you needed support in the past, now you can offer it to

someone else. No one can relate to what a cancer patient is going through better than a cancer survivor.

The network of cancer survivors is strong and extensive. In fact, the National Cancer Survivors Day Foundation (www.ncsdf.org) sponsors an annual event to celebrate life after cancer. The event served as the inspiration for the creation of the National Cancer Institute's Office of Cancer Survivorship (OCS) in 1996.

To find survivor support groups or connect with other cancer survivors, visit the following Web sites.

- Cancer Survivors Online: www.cancer survivors.org
- Lung Cancer Alliance: www.alcase.org (on the home page, click on "Support Programs")
- University of Texas M.D. Anderson Cancer Center: www.mdanderson.org (on the home page, click on "Support Programs" under the "For Patients and Public" tab)

For Your Life

As much as you may be looking forward to reconnecting with friends and reestablishing your social life, you need to go slowly at first. Everyone will understand if you make short nights of your initial outings. In fact, they will understand if you'd prefer that they visit you at your home, rather than you schlepping out to see them. Later, as you feel up to it, you may go out more. The key is to not overdo. Pay attention to your physical comfort level, as well as your emotional state. These will give you a true reading on what you're capable of doing and how soon.

The same rule applies if you're planning to return to work. Yes, it's one of the quickest ways to get back in the swing of things once you've completed treatment. It also may be the fastest route to stress that you really could do without right now. Before you head back to your workplace, it might be wise to arrange a meeting with your boss. The two of you can discuss a schedule that will allow you to ease into your job. Perhaps you can start half-days, with the understanding that you will need to gauge your energy level for the first couple of weeks. You also might mention that you may be taking time off for doctors' appointments, physical therapy, or counseling sessions.

Then again, rather than immersing yourself in your job or your social life, you might be thinking about getting away from the constant reminders of your illness—even the loved ones who have stood by you through your treatment. If you feel like escaping, escape.

The question is, are you up to travel? The key factors, as always, are your physical comfort level and your emotional state. No matter how important a trip may seem, you must measure its importance against the discomfort you may feel during and especially after your trip. Perhaps you won't know until you've tested the waters—or the air or the roads or whatever your means of transportation. If you find that you've bitten off more than you can chew, don't starve yourself. Just take smaller bites. The following strategies can help ensure smooth travel.

- Stock a small cooler with snacks and beverages.
- Take along books and tapes to help pass the time.
- Pack your cell phone.
- Tell several people of your travel plans.
- Know where to find medical services en route. A good resource is the International Association for Medical Assistance to Travellers, which can direct you to medical care anywhere in the world. To learn more, visit www.iamat.org.
- Plan to do less than you normally would on your trips.
- Try to find a way to sit that allows you to stretch out.
- Schedule an appointment with a massage therapist. These days, many hotels offer massage and other spa-type services on-site. If not, the concierge may be able to refer you to a qualified massage therapist nearby.

REVIEW LONG-TERM PLANS

Back in Step 3, we suggested doing some advance planning by collecting information on maintenance protocols that support remission and help prevent recurrence. Of course, since you've just completed treatment, probably the farthest thing from your mind is more treatment. But you should take this opportunity to review the information and to discuss your options with your treating oncologist or your cancer patient advocate (if you have one). They can advise you on the best course of action in light of what they know about your cancer as well as available protocols.

If vaccine therapy was an option for your cancer, you would have needed to bank diseased tissue for use in preparing the vaccine. Now you should ask your treating oncologist whether you are a candidate for any of the ongoing vaccine trials, as it may require additional planning at this juncture. The two of you can obtain up-to-date information on eligibility requirements and other pertinent information, so you can make a decision on whether to enter a trial—and which one.

Other maintenance protocols are in various stages of development. For example, scientists are testing an array of natural and synthetic substances that have shown promise in preventing or delaying a recurrence of cancer. Among the so-called chemopreventives to successfully emerge from clinical trial is tamoxifen (Nolvadex). It earned FDA approval in 1998 as an effective breast cancer preventive. Tamoxifen belongs to a class of chemopreventive substances called blocking agents, which include flavonoids, indoles, isothiocyanates, and oltipraz. The other class is suppressing agents—among them calcium, vitamin A and the retinoids, and vitamin D and related compounds, as well as aspirin and other nonsteroidal anti-inflammatory drugs (NSAIDs).

If you recruited a national expert or a research medical oncologist for your medical team, ask that person for updates on any clinical trials you may have come across during your initial search in Step 3. Also good resources are organizations dedicated to your specific type of cancer, such as the Leukemia and Lymphoma Society and the Lung Cancer Alliance. Don't forget to ask other cancer survivors and to check online for additional leads.

Keep in mind that for many clinical trials, eligibility is determined by the requirements of the grants that are funding the trials. Their mission is to serve the greater good rather than the needs of individual patients.

DEAL WITH RECURRENCE

What if, despite your best efforts, your cancer comes back? You have a number of options at your disposal and a number of decisions to make. It will require significant strength, courage, and hope, as well as every ounce of confidence, commitment, and faith that you can muster. You may need to dig even deeper than before.

In consultation with your treating oncologist and other members of your medical team, you should weigh the benefits and risks of continuing your current treatment regimen or trying something different. You could look at it as an opportunity to start over. Perhaps new or experimental protocols are available that weren't before. You could choose to pursue a more aggressive therapy . . . or to do nothing at all.

The decision is yours, and it isn't an easy one. Essentially, you're weighing the possibility of cure against the reality of treatment—a reality that you know all too well. Modern medicine is wondrous for its ability to extend life. But at some point, you must ask, at what price?

PCMS Tool #7.2: Assess Quality of Life Markers

As you consider your options for dealing with recurrence, your quality of life will carry considerable weight in your decision-making process. From previous exercises, you probably have some sense of what "quality of life" means to you. The worksheet on page 160 provides more concrete markers against which to gauge your options and determine which path is most appropriate for you.

For each of the 17 markers—14 that reflect psychological/emotional well-being, 3 for physical well-being—consider its value in what you would define as a satisfactory quality of life. Then circle the corresponding rating between 1 and 10. Generally, those markers with ratings to the left of the center line are more important to you, while those with ratings to the right of the center line are less likely to compromise your quality of life.

Decide What's Next

Using the above-mentioned worksheet for reference, you and your treating oncologist can have a meaningful conversation about next steps. Compare each of your options against your ideal quality of life, as revealed by your scores for all the markers. Through this process, some options will rise to the top, while others will fall away. Here's what's on the table.

Investigate experimental protocols and your

eligibility for them. Again, the specifics of your cancer will determine whether or not you qualify for one of these protocols. Just don't let the word *experimental* frighten you. Remember, almost every treatment that's in use now had to prove itself in clinical trials first.

The more information you gather about clinical trials, the more confidence you'll have in choosing one. Ask lots of questions of your cancer patient advocate and/or your national expert or research medical oncologist. Be sure to find out whether any new trials have launched since you originally did your research.

The Coalition of Cancer Cooperative Groups maintains a list of clinical trials. For information, call (877) 520-4457 or visit the organization's Web site at www.cancertrials help.org.

Explore alternatives to conventional medicine. If you go this route, be aware that you may not get much support from your treating oncologist or from other members of your medical team. Talk through your decision with your cancer patient advocate or with your therapist, counselor, or mental health professional. You'll need to fortify yourself against those who will criticize your decision and try to persuade you to change your mind.

It's important to not see alternative therapies as a last-ditch, desperate attempt—the proverbial Hail Mary pass in football. Your willingness to explore all options, even those beyond the realm of conventional medicine, is a sign of strength and confidence. If a therapy fails, you can feel good that you left no stoned unturned, and you can move on with pride.

Do nothing and come to acceptance. You may

PCMS Tool #7.2

QUALITY OF LIFE MARKERS

Drive	1 2 3 4 5	6 7 8 9 10	Lack of interest
Laughter/joy	1 2 3 4 5	6 7 8 9 10	Blues/depression
Fun	1 2 3 4 5	6 7 8 9 10	Boredom
Happiness	1 2 3 4 5	6 7 8 9 10	Sadness
Health	1 2 3 4 5	6 7 8 9 10	Illness
Pleasure	1 2 3 4 5	6 7 8 9 10	Dissatisfaction
Adventure	1 2 3 4 5	6 7 8 9 10	Fear
Vitality	1 2 3 4 5	6 7 8 9 10	Lethargy
Peace	1 2 3 4 5	6 7 8 9 10	Confusion
Contentment	1 2 3 4 5	6 7 8 9 10	Discontent
Rewarding	1 2 3 4 5	6 7 8 9 10	Unfulfilling
Productive	1 2 3 4 5	6 7 8 9 10	Useless
Surprising	1 2 3 4 5	6 7 8 9 10	Predictable
Challenging	1 2 3 4 5	6 7 8 9 10	Overwhelming
Pain-free	1 2 3 4 5	6 7 8 9 10	Pain
Nausea-free	1 2 3 4 5	6 7 8 9 10	Nausea
Energetic	1 2 3 4 5	6 7 8 9 10	Fatigue

conclude that enough is enough. More treatment will only bring more pain, and you don't see any value in lowering your quality of life to such a degree. You can do no more and no better. This is not defeat; it's acceptance. Doing nothing could be one of the most positive and proactive statements of your life. It all depends on your attitude.

Once you make the decision to do nothing, you still have much to do. Make the most of the weeks or months you have left. There are personal matters and paperwork to organize, trips to take, and—most important—people to see, with whom to spend quality time and to share things that you may have been holding back. For a complete discussion of issues to think about and plan for, see Steps 9 and 10 (pages 177 and 183).

Proactively end your life. One of modern medicine's most controversial issues is euthanasia. Choosing to end your life when the pain and suffering are no longer endurable is the most personal decision you can make. In our opinion, the decision is so personal that no one—not your spouse or children, not your treating oncologist, not your spiritual counselor—can or should advise you on it. Yes, they can share their feelings and opinions, and yes, you probably will consider their feelings and opinions as you make up your mind. But in the end, it is up to you and you alone.

Saar considered this option early in the cancer process. He discussed it with me and our children at our first meeting together. He had a very workable plan, and he was ready to put it into place. Later he wrote, "I have felt for years that when the treatment curve going upward crosses the quality of life curve going downward, then it is time to rethink further treatment objectives." When asked if he had the courage to take action, he said that he did. And he was right.

If you would like more information, visit the following Web sites.

- John D. Thompson Hospice Institute: www.hospice.com
- National Hospice and Palliative Care Organization: www.nhpco.org

FEELING GRATITUDE

When Saar went into remission, he looked toward the future and dared to ask himself: "What do I want to do with the rest of my life?" He felt that writing about his frame of mind at this miraculous point in his life might help set his path. As he wrote in his journal:

I was attending the "Leadership at the Peak" course at the Center for Creative Leadership in Colorado Springs. The CCL is a nonprofit think tank that provides leadership training and feedback for executives and managers. Over the 5 days of the course, the 12 members of our group had bonded as we shared our lives, our experiences, and our hopes for the future.

The last morning of the course was to be a "goal setting" session. Goal setting is a common exercise to induce people to use what they've learned to change their behavior—hopefully for the better. The assignment was to write a letter to ourselves, which would be mailed to us in 6 months, to see if we had done what we said we would do.

I listened attentively as the first seven of my colleagues read off their letters. The VP at General Motors, the three-star general, the insurance executive, and the others all gave honest appraisals of what they hoped to accomplish in the workplace and in their personal lives. Then it was my turn.

I was somewhat reluctant to share my letter with the group. I felt that my comments were very personal and may not be appropriate, as they were not in line with the business at hand. I began by explaining that I had written many such letters previously—10 years, 5 years, 3 years before this one. With each letter, I had meant to do what I said I would do. More often than not, I failed to set priorities, and many of the goals went unmet. I urged the group to set priorities. I urged them to put things into proper perspective, and that didn't mean business first.

Then I began to read:

"Dear Saar,

"If you are reading this letter, it means you have reached . . .

"Goal 1—you are alive. I hope that you are still in remission and reasonable health. Did the nutrition, exercise, and meditation programs you started and promised to follow through with help to get rid of the cancer fatigue? I wish you could tell me now what worked, and when, so I could feel less anxious and frustrated.

"Goal 2—pursue other rehabilitation programs, physical and cognitive, that you started and promised to finish. Did you gain back your losses? Did you learn new coping skills?

"Now let's focus on some of the more specific goals you discussed at CCL.

"Goal 3—move along toward a new career or occupation. Have you decided what to do and how? Did you decide on medicine, consulting, or something else? I figured that you would synthesize many tasks—teaching, writing, and consulting—to create that exciting business you wanted to establish.

"Did you add, as you always have, food for your soul, the community work you love? Is the new program you wanted to start at the Los Angeles Free Clinic—on Alternative Methods of Managing Menopause—up and running?

"Have you written the book proposal you promised by December? Was it accepted, revised, or discarded? With so many titles and topics bouncing around in your head, you acted more like an indecisive type than what you are: the judgmental type who gets things done.

"Goal 4—get your golf handicap back down to 16 or less. Are the balls still going straight, or has your slice returned? Last August, you were hitting your 4 iron off the tee and averaging 195 yards. It seemed the sicker you were, the easier you swung, and the farther and straighter the ball went.

"Goal 5—spend more quality and getting-away time with Toni. Have you replanned the trip to Scotland that you were supposed to take with her, then had to cancel because the cancer got in the way? Do you still go out for a date one night a week? Do you still tell her you love her, and how much you appreciate her, at least five times a week?

"There are so many other goals to set, but to be realistic, if you have accomplished these, you will have come a long way. There are so many changes happening to you—changes in how you see the world, how you speak, how you treat others. Have you expanded on this newer, softer side of you?

"And, finally, have you been in touch with any of the guys from CCL? There was such warm and wonderful camaraderie in your group. Did Marty get his blood pressure down; Bill, his weight down; and Madison, his cholesterol? If you don't know, shame on you. You cared then, why not now?

—Saar"

DIVISION OF LABOR

TASK	WHO WILL DO IT		
	YOU	PERSONAL ADVOCATE	CPA
1. Celebrate being alive.			
2. Photocopy and complete the values and goals assessments in PCMS Tool #7.1.			
3. Implement self-care strategies to support your recovery.			
4. Review long-term plans.			
5. If you experience a recurrence, weigh your options against your quality of life markers (PCMS Tool #7.2).			

STEP 8

ADDRESS LEGAL AND FINANCIAL ISSUES

Rabbi and Anna Silverstein had been happily married for 50 years when Anna became very ill. On her deathbed, Anna once again declared her love for her husband and told him what a wonderful partner he had been. The rabbi, with tears in his eyes, said to his wife, "I love you. You have made me so happy. We are both old, and I know I will join you very soon. Then, we will be together unto all eternity." Anna smiled, held his hand, and passed away peacefully.

Rabbi Silverstein was not the same after that. He took to walking around the house muttering, "What to do, what to do?" His children became very worried about him. Finally, his son asked what was wrong. The rabbi replied, "I promised your mother that I would join her in heaven." "So?" asked his son. "Suppose I don't go to heaven!" shouted his father. "I haven't given enough money to the temple and to the poor. Quick, call a lawyer. I need to set up a charitable trust to make donations. Then I can keep my promise to my beloved Anna."

Even Rabbi Silverstein understood the importance of putting his affairs in order before it was too late to control his destiny. Financial paperwork such as doctor and hospital bills, insurance claims, and prescriptions must be organized and processed while you're able to think clearly. So, too, must legal matters—checking your will, preparing an advance directive. Of course, none of these tasks is especially pleasant. But if you deal with them promptly, early in your illness, you won't attach as much emotion to them. Then you will be able to put your energy into what's most important: your health.

As soon as possible after diagnosis, you should decide who you want as your legal and financial representatives. An attorney and an accountant are natural choices. Make clear to them what you want them to do. Among the three of you, you should cover all of the following points.

DELEGATE LEGAL AUTHORITY

In the event that you would become unable to make decisions about your medical care, you can spell out your wishes yourself or appoint another person to act on your behalf. This would be done in a document known as an advance directive.

Under the Patient Self-Determination Act, which became law in 1991, hospitals that receive Medicare or Medicaid funding must advise patients of their right to execute advance directives. Since then, all 50 states have passed their own laws recognizing advance directives as binding legal documents, though regulation of them varies from one state to the next.

The term *advance directive* actually applies

to two types of legal documents: a living will and a medical power of attorney.

Living will: This document sets forth instructions about which medical treatments you want and don't want at the end of life. Its purpose is to guide your physician and family in deciding how aggressively to pursue measures that would delay death. A living will also may go by one of the following names: a directive to physicians, a health care declaration, or a medical directive.

Medical power of attorney: This document identifies the person you want to make medical decisions for you once you no longer can do so yourself. In some states, it may be known as a durable power of attorney for health care, an appointment of a health care agent, or a health care proxy.

At minimum, your advance directive will spell out your wishes for three procedures that may become necessary at some point in your care: ventilator-assisted breathing; feeding tube; and CPR, including defibrillation. It isn't an all-or-nothing arrangement. You may feel comfortable with one of the procedures but not the rest, and so can choose accordingly.

You don't need to consult an attorney in order to draft an advance directive. You can obtain sample documents from your attorney or your state health department. Computer software packages also are available; just be sure that you use the document templates for your state. Otherwise, the advance directive may not be valid.

Keep in mind that in some states, an advance directive is not valid when a patient is pregnant or once paramedics have been called. Then the emergency personnel are required to do what is necessary to stabilize the patient for transfer to a hospital.

While we're on the subject, we want to mention another document called a "do not resuscitate" order, or DNR. Unlike living wills and medical power of attorneys, DNRs cannot be prepared by patients. A patient can request one, but his or her doctor must sign it in order to make it legal.

A DNR order stops the administration of CPR. As you may know, CPR is an emergency medical intervention that circulates blood and oxygen to vital organs in the absence of spontaneous breathing and cardiac rhythm. Hospitals and paramedics will administer CPR unless they have on file a physician's order to withhold treatment.

PCMS Tool #8.1: Anticipate End-of-Life Care

Attorney Jim Towey—a former legal advisor to Mother Teresa and founder of the nonprofit organization Aging with Dignity—developed Five Wishes, an eight-page form that serves as a legally binding advance directive in 34 states and the District of Columbia. Written in plain language and easy to use, the form guides readers through these key questions surrounding end-of-life care.

- Who do I want to make health-care decisions for me when I can't?

- What kind of medical treatment do I want or don't want?

- What would help me feel comfortable while I am dying?

- How do I want people to treat me?

- What do I want my loved ones to know about me after I'm gone?

For a copy of *Five Wishes*, send a $5 check or money order to Aging with Dignity, P.O. Box 1661, Tallahassee, FL 32302-1661. Orders from Florida must add sales tax. To place your order online, visit www.agingwithdignity.org.

Discussing Your Wishes

Often patients are reluctant to execute advance directives and DNRs, perhaps subconsciously believing that doing so could hasten their deaths. Having delayed his own paperwork, Saar wrote, "These are steps that should be taken and revised when people are well, not just when they're anticipating death."

Another important point: Advance directives are only as useful as the personal communication to support them. No document could cover every situation or circumstance. You must reinforce your advance directives by explaining your views of medical care and quality of life to the physicians and loved ones who will participate in the decision-making process.

The most important of these conversations is the one with the person chosen as your designate (sometimes known as a proxy or surrogate). It's critical to pick someone who's willing to take on the responsibility of carrying out your wishes, even if that person doesn't necessarily agree with them. Your best bet may be your spouse or partner. If you appoint someone from outside the family, such as your attorney, find out whether the person could encounter any legal challenges, should family members disagree with their decisions.

Once your designate is onboard, your next step is to call together your family and friends to inform them of your wishes. Your loved ones may assume that you're giving up and urge that you change your mind. Allowing them to express their concerns now may help stave off dissent later. Make clear that you're presenting this information while you still have the mental faculties to do so. Then if you ever become unable to make your own decisions, your designate can step in and act on your behalf, relieving the burden from everyone else.

PCMS Tool #8.2: Practice What You Want to Say

If you aren't quite sure how to broach the topic of end-of-life care with your loved ones, or you simply are looking for pointers to guide your conversation, we've prepared the following script for reference. You don't need to read it word for word; rather, use it as a jumping-off point, tailoring the comments to your particular situation.

Welcome, and thank you for coming. I know this conversation might be uncomfortable for some of you, as it is for me. But I think it's necessary, and in the end, it will make things easier for all of us. I will feel better knowing that I've already made some important decisions and won't need to deal with them when I'm in severe pain or not clearheaded. I think you will feel better if you know what my wishes are and who is going to be responsible for taking action when I cannot.

As you must have gathered by now, I need

help. I need someone to be the project manager, the person who takes charge and oversees the tasks that we're going to discuss here. I need someone who feels able to demand more morphine or request hospice care or even pull the plug—whatever I have decided I want to happen. I need someone who's objective enough to follow through on my requests without letting emotions get in the way, and compassionate enough to act with as much sensitivity as possible. I need someone who can think rationally in the midst of emotional crisis. I need someone I trust, someone I expect will be healthy and alive when the time comes. After much thought, I have decided that [person's name here] should represent me.

I called all of you here because I want to explain my wishes in person. Though I've made my choices, I want to hear your thoughts and feelings. I'm sure there are issues that I've not considered and that you can help bring to light. In turn, I may have questions for you, which I hope you will answer as best as you can.

Some of you may disagree with whom I have chosen to be my designate and the guidelines that I have given him [or her]. It is important to me that everyone understand and respect my designate's responsibility for following through on my requests. If all of us agree on this now, we can avoid any conflict or questioning of authority down the road. Does each of you accept this? Are you willing to abide by my wishes, even if you object to them? If not, please say so now, so we can work through the issues you raise. I am open to discussion, but not to changing who is to be my designate.

I'm doing this so none of you has to make difficult decisions during what most certainly will be a highly stressful time. You're here be-cause I love you and because you have stood by me throughout my illness. I want your arms around me now and to the end.

Keeping Track of Your Advance Directive

Given all the confusion surrounding a serious illness such as cancer, it isn't surprising that as many as 35 percent of advance directives cannot be found when they're needed. So this doesn't happen to you, be sure to:

- Give copies of all advance directive documents—including the medical power of attorney—to your designate as well as to your doctor, hospital, personal advocate, and one or two loved ones. Tell them where you're keeping the original documents (not in a safe deposit box, which they may not be able to access until after your death).

- If you have more than one residence, register your advance directives with the hospitals in each location. You also might want to consider naming more than one designate, so you have someone to speak for you wherever you might be.

- Carry copies in your purse, wallet, or briefcase or in the glove compartment of your car.

- Register your living will and medical power of attorney with the US Living Will Registry either online at www.us livingwillregistry.com or by phone at (800) 548-9455. This free, confidential service will instantly fax copies of the documents to your hospital upon request. It also will send reminders to update the documents as necessary.

ORGANIZE YOUR FINANCIAL AFFAIRS

Just as you've chosen someone to speak on your behalf regarding health care decisions, you may want to appoint someone to manage your legal and financial affairs if you aren't able to do so. This person has what's known as legal power of attorney. Your legal designate can be—and, according to some experts, should be—someone other than your medical designate.

Depending on the complexity of your personal finances, you also might consider enlisting the services of an accountant, a business manager, an investment broker, an insurance agent, and/or an attorney. Collectively, they can help organize your wills, trusts, insurance policies, and other estate planning documents. They also can keep track of your income and expenses—from checking and savings accounts, IRAs, and real estate holdings to medical bills, car payments, and mortgages.

If you prefer to manage your own finances, then you should set aside a day for collecting all of the paperwork that represents your full financial worth. Estimate what you own, what you owe, and what you could liquidate if necessary. Then write down this information, make copies of the relevant documents, and review all the materials with your legal designate.

Many months into treatment, Saar realized that he would need to sell his practice. The high-dose chemotherapy was draining his energy. With the knowledge of what was to come and the likelihood of not being able to handle the high volume of patients and the many hours of physical activity, he put out feelers for a buyer. He was determined to find someone who would not only meet his asking price but also deliver customized, empathic, expert breast health care.

After he discovered that the most interested buyer was stringing out negotiations, hoping to lower the price as Saar became weaker, he got more aggressive about courting the other candidates. Eventually, he chose one—Lawrence Resnick, MD. And he learned a valuable lesson. As he wrote:

I realized early on that I could and would be my worst enemy in negotiations. I should not have been representing myself—as no one in my condition should do. One of my closest friends, Lee Weisel, stepped up to the plate and took over for me. Lee was the negotiator, working with another dear friend and attorney, Ross Arbiter, to make the best possible deal for me. Thank goodness for that team. They made sure that my patients would be happy and well taken care of; that my loyal staff (some of whom had been with me for 10 years) and wonderful office manager, Anna, also would taken care of; and that I would be able to get on with my treatments, which by then had become a full-time job.

When we are physically ill and concerned about staying alive, we are not capable of negotiating contracts to our advantage. You should

find someone to act as your advocate in business deals, just as you found someone to be your advocate in your cancer fight. Trying to be a macho man or a superwoman, and prove that you are still able when you may not be, is foolish. When you need help, get help.

For more information on the financial issues that can affect cancer patients, refer to the "Financial and Legal Matters" section of the American Cancer Society Web site: www.cancer.org (from the home page, click "Patients, Family, and Friends," then "Coping with Treatment," then "Managing Day to Day").

EVALUATE YOUR INSURANCE COVERAGE

With a serious illness such as cancer, the cost of care can add up rather quickly. If you are employed outside the home, a group health plan may pick up the tab for your medical expenses. At minimum, a good group policy will cover a portion of the diagnostic tests, as well as the treatment itself.

These days, many employers choose health maintenance organizations or preferred provider organizations over traditional health coverage. Both have their pros and cons.

Health maintenance organizations (HMOs): Like other health insurance, most HMOs require a minimal co-payment, reimbursing the provider for the remaining cost. Because most HMOs require providers to enter into contracts by which they agree to accept reduced fees for their services, you may be limited in your choice of physicians. Some HMOs offer an "out of network" option, which allows you to consult the doctor of your choice. Then you must pay the difference between the HMO's in-network reimbursement and the doctor's fees. HMOs also may require a referral from your primary care practitioner to any specialist in order to qualify for reimbursement.

Preferred provider organizations (PPOs): Compared with HMOs, PPOs tend to offer broader health benefits, with more choice in providers, procedures, and prescription drugs. Many PPOs allow patients to consult specialists without referrals from their primary care practitioners and to go out of network at will (what's known as a point of service option). Providers who belong to PPOs generally can charge what they consider a fair fee for service, which means that you're responsible for the difference between the PPO's reimbursement rate and the doctor's fee.

Most hospitals, cancer centers, and doctors' offices have someone on staff who specializes in health insurance benefits and can decipher what your policy will and will not pay for. This person may be able to assist in filling out complicated insurance claim forms. Another option is to hire an independent financial manager who has experience handling insurance claims. Coming from outside the system, this person would represent your interests—not the hospital's, the doctor's, or the insurer's. Should you need to resolve billing disputes or make payment arrangements, your financial manager can intervene on your behalf.

If you have private health insurance—say, because you own a business or are otherwise self-employed—your insurance agent or broker should be able to address any questions about your policy.

- Which benefits in your policy are specific to cancer diagnosis and treatment?

- Do these benefits have a cap?

- Does your policy exclude anything that you should be aware of?

- Do you have adequate coverage, given your age and current health status?

- How do your policy's benefits and premiums compare with those of other insurance companies?

- Do you have the best coverage for what you need and can afford?

Some insurers offer what's known as a catastrophic illness clause as an add-on to their health insurance policies. It kicks in after you've exhausted your other benefits, so you aren't left to pay medical expenses out of pocket. Check whether your plan contains this provision.

No matter what the source of your health insurance, you'll find that the paperwork from all the bills and claims can pile up quickly. To help stay on top of it, we suggest the following organizational strategies:

- File claims for all medical expenses, even when you aren't sure that your policy covers a particular item.

- Submit claims as you receive them. Don't risk missing a deadline buried in fine print.

- Make copies of all paperwork related to your claims, such as letters to doctors, hospitals, insurance companies, and other relevant people and institutions. Also make copies of bills, receipts, and requests for sick leave.

- Keep an accurate record of all claims submitted, pending, and paid.

- Don't let your medical insurance expire. Pay your premiums in full and on time. Once you've had a major illness such as cancer, getting new coverage can be difficult.

Government-Sponsored Health Coverage

If you have no health insurance, you may qualify for federal assistance. Don't be too proud or embarrassed to apply. Such programs exist for just this purpose.

Medicare: Medicare is a federally run group health plan for those over age 65 or permanently disabled and therefore eligible for Social Security Insurance (SSI) benefits. Anyone who has been collecting SSI payments for at least 24 months is entitled to Medicare benefits as well.

Medicare health insurance has two parts. Part A provides reimbursement for hospital care, home health care, hospice care, and Medicare-certified nursing facilities. Part B covers physicians' services, diagnostic tests, certain home medical equipment, and ambulance use.

If your HMO has a contract with Medicare, it must offer the same medical benefits as Medicare. In turn, you must use your HMO's network of providers.

Medicare is a good source of basic health coverage, but it has its limitations. If you have any questions about eligibility or benefits, you can contact Medicare by phone at (800) 633-4227 or online at www.medicare.gov. Another good resource is the Health Insurance Counseling and Advocacy Program (HICAP), a joint federal/state program that provides information and assistance on Medicare, along with other types of health insurance. The New York State office has posted links to other states' programs through its Web site: www.hiicap.state.ny.us (click on "Help Links," then on "Help in Other States").

Medigap: You can expand your Medicare benefits with what's known as a Medigap policy. There are 10 types of policies, designated by letters A through J. Each one offers a different mix of benefits; those that include prescription drug coverage carry the highest premiums.

Medicaid: To be eligible for Medicaid, your total income and assets must fall below a certain level, which differs from state to state. Some providers do not accept Medicaid. For more information, contact your state's Medicaid office.

Medical assistance programs: Some hospitals that receive funding from the federal government must sponsor Hill-Burton Free Care Programs, which provide free or low-cost health care to those who are unable to pay. The Health Resources and Services Administration (HRSA) has established a hotline to address questions about the Hill-Burton pro-

Colin's Coverage

Colin had been a healthy guy—maybe a little overweight, maybe drank a little too much, but without any real medical issues. Then at age 55, he found out he had prostate cancer. As he investigated the available treatments, he decided on the newest type of surgery, which would preserve his nerves and give him the best chance of remaining sexually potent as well as continent. Unfortunately, his HMO considered the procedure experimental and wouldn't pay for it.

Colin was running out of time. Not willing to risk incontinence and impotence when he didn't have to, he went ahead with the procedure and paid for it himself.

Several months after he recovered and felt stronger, he tried to get the insurance company to pay. They refused, using innumerable tactics to stall the claim. Finally, Colin hired a cancer patient advocate who specialized in contract and insurance issues to challenge the insurance company. Working together, they discovered loop-holes in the insurance contract and won their case. Six months after he started working with the advocate, Colin collected his money.

Had Colin known in advance that his insurance wouldn't pay for many of the more expensive procedures for more serious illnesses, he might have done several things differently. For example, he could have chosen a more expensive health plan with better benefits. He could have switched insurance companies when he turned 50. He could have challenged his insurance company far enough in advance to build a case before surgery. Or he could have taken out cancer insurance, which would have covered his surgery.

All of us can learn from Colin's experience. Dealing with financial and legal issues can seem overwhelming—but *not* dealing with them is worse. The ultimate proactive act is to look squarely at your real-life circumstances and take action so that you don't become a victim.

gram; call (800) 638-0742 or (800) 492-0359 for Maryland residents. The HRSA Web site also posts a list of facilities that offer health care services under the program. The direct link is http://www.hrsa.gov/osp/dfcr/about/aboutdiv.htm.

Veterans' benefits: If you are a veteran, you may qualify for special health benefits. For the most up-to-date information, consult the Web site for the Veterans Benefits Administration: www.vba.va.gov.

Life Insurance

If you have a life insurance policy, you may be able to collect on the death benefit while you're living through what's known as a viatical, or life, settlement. Essentially, you sell your policy to a third party for more than its cash surrender value but less than its death benefit. While you can use this money to cover medical expenses, you must keep in mind that (1) your heirs won't be able to collect anything from the policy and (2) the viatical may not be reversible.

Viaticals fall under the jurisdiction of state insurance departments. To learn more about this option, visit the Web site for the Viatical and Life Settlement Association of America: www.viatical.org. The site includes information by state.

Disability Insurance

As mentioned earlier, people who become permanently disabled before age 65 may be eligible for payments under the federal SSI program. To find out whether you would qualify, your best resource is the Social Security Administration Web site: www.ssa.gov. On the home page, click on "Disability and SSI." The site includes a screening tool to assess eligibility, as well as an online form to apply for benefits.

Beyond the SSI program, many states offer limited disability payments through private employers. Your employer may offer its own disability benefits. For more information, contact your company's benefits officer or human resources representative. Be sure to find out the terms of the disability coverage, including how much per month you're entitled to receive and for how many months.

Also inquire about other possible compensation for your illness, such as payment for unused sick days or vacation days.

RESOLVE WORKPLACE DISPUTES

The Americans with Disabilities Act expressly prohibits employers from discriminating against employees who are ill. Until recently, though, cancer patients and cancer survivors have had relatively few legitimate resources for legal advice specific to their condition. To fill the gap, Loyola Law School and the Western Law Center for Disability Rights joined forces to establish the Cancer Legal Resource Center, which offers confidential counseling on cancer-related legal issues. If you have a specific question, you can call the center at (213) 736-1455. For general information, go to http://wlcdr.everybody. org/; under "Services," click on Legal Representation, then on "Cancer Legal Resource Center."

Another good resource is the Patient Advocate Foundation, which serves as a liaison between patients and their employers to resolve workplace issues that have arisen from the patients' diagnoses. To learn more, visit the foundation's Web site at www.patient advocate.org, which features the downloadable guide "First My Illness . . . Now Job Discrimination: Steps to Resolution." (From the home page, click on "Resources," then on "PAF Publications.")

Division of Labor

TASK	WHO WILL DO IT		
	YOU	PERSONAL ADVOCATE	CPA
1. Draft a living will.			
2. Appoint a medical power of attorney.			
3. Discuss your wishes for end-of-life care with your loved ones.			
4. Consult your financial advisor or another appropriate expert about your personal finances.			
5. Take care of any necessary business transactions.			
6. Find out what your health insurance will and won't cover.			
7. If you don't have health insurance, explore your eligibility for government-sponsored health benefits.			
8. Tell your employer how much you can contribute and what you will need from him or her.			

STEP 9

UNDERSTAND PALLIATIVE CARE

In the past, *palliative care* was something of a code phrase for "We've lost the fight." It referred to what was done for patients for whom treatment wasn't working, for whom remission or cure wasn't possible, or for whom the only goal was to be as comfortable and pain free as possible through the last stage of life.

Today, however, palliative care is part of the conversation from the outset of cancer treatment, because of the enlightened view that a patient's comfort should be a consideration all along. With its growing importance, palliative care—much like pain management—has evolved into a highly sophisticated medical specialty.

Palliative care aims at providing comfort by controlling or managing physical, psychological, emotional, and spiritual suffering. In other words, it considers the needs of the whole patient. As such, it is serving a much broader range of cancer patients who could benefit from such measures at an earlier stage of the disease process.

Let's say someone with colon cancer has reached a point in treatment where he and his doctor agree that he cannot achieve a cure. He may opt to continue chemotherapy to extend his life and to improve his quality of life, by reducing the size of his tumor and providing relief from pain. For this patient, the treatment is the same as when a cure was the goal. Only now, its purpose is to relieve symptoms and prevent complications.

Patients and their doctors may choose to shift from curative to palliative care for a number of reasons. As in the example above, the cancer may not be responding to curative measures, and so the patient and doctor need to rethink the goal of treatment. Perhaps the side effects of treatment are more than the patient can tolerate. Or maybe treatment is undermining quality of life to a degree that the patient finds unacceptable.

The most difficult part of palliative care is deciding when it has become necessary. At this critical point in the cancer process, it is important to talk with your treating oncologist, your personal advocate and (if you have one) professional cancer advocate, and your loved ones. Then you need to spend some time alone, to be introspective.

Some family members and friends, and even some doctors, may say that you're giving up by shifting from finding a cure to extending life or simply finding peace of mind. Only you can make that decision. And only you need to feel comfortable with the decision.

THE ADVANTAGES OF PALLIATIVE CARE

Every cancer patient has a unique response to treatment, as well as to side effects. With pal-

liative care, the patient's individual needs—as well as the type and stage of cancer—get full consideration in formulating a treatment plan.

Among the most important functions of palliative care is to provide effective pain management. Remember that while pain often accompanies cancer and its treatment, you don't need to suffer through it. Health care practitioners who specialize in palliative care know the latest pain management techniques, from medication and surgery to alternative and complementary therapies. With all of these options at their disposal, practitioners can design a program to alleviate your particular pain.

That said, you do need to be proactive. You should become as knowledgeable as possible about your symptoms and the available treatments, so you're able to articulate them and get the relief you're seeking. Often cancer patients are so anxious or upset that they aren't able to clearly verbalize how they're feeling. Fortunately, palliative caregivers are expert listeners. They learn to sift through a patient's concerns in a very systematic way, so they can provide appropriate care.

This outreach extends to the patient's family as well. Palliative caregivers will encourage loved ones to ask questions and to share in decision making. If a family member is struggling to cope with the situation, the palliative caregiver can offer comfort and counseling.

Your Palliative Care Team

As mentioned earlier, palliative care addresses the physical, emotional, and spiritual needs of the cancer patient. For the body, a typical caregiving plan might focus on alleviating pain, nausea, fatigue, and other symptoms, whether brought on by the cancer or by its treatment. For the mind and spirit, palliative care can help overcome anxiety and depression and lift morale, often by providing a fresh perspective on the disease process itself.

Befitting its whole-patient philosophy, palliative care typically combines conventional medicine with complementary and alternative therapies such as acupuncture, energy healing, and medication. In all likelihood, your caregiving team will consist of health care practitioners from many disciplines. Some hospitals have palliative care specialists on staff who can coordinate your team for you. You may want to seek out your own practitioners, so that you aren't dealing with the economic constraints of the managed care hospital environment. Plus, you'll have greater flexibility in the event that you receive care at home.

Your personal advocate and cancer patient advocate can help recruit qualified practitioners for your palliative care team. Its members might include any or all of the following:

- Primary care physician

- Treating oncologist

- Pain management specialist

- Physical and occupational therapists

- Pharmacist

- Nurse

- Home health aide

- CAM practitioners

- Psycho-oncologist (a mental health professional who has special training to work with cancer patients)

- Clergy

HOSPICE CARE

Hospice provides palliative care for patients as they approach the end of life. These are people who no longer can benefit from curative measures. Their doctors have confirmed that their life expectancy is 6 months or less.

Hospice services are available in various settings—at home, in hospitals and skilled nursing facilities, and in special hospice centers. As with general palliative care, a typical hospice team includes health care professionals from various disciplines, including doctors, nurses, psychologists, social workers, clergy, bereavement specialists, and CAM practitioners. Volunteers provide critical support as well.

Among the primary purposes of hospice is to manage pain and other symptoms, so the patient can remain alert and comfortable. Hospice also can be enormously helpful in dealing with the psychological and/or spiritual crises that are common among those with terminal illnesses. While hospice professionals can't erase all the distress, they lend a welcome ear or shoulder to patients who don't wish to burden loved ones with concerns and fears at such a stressful time.

Those who work in hospice programs also have special training to deal with bereavement, which can be invaluable not just

Sixty-year-old Casey thought that his stage I melanoma had been cured. Eight years after his original diagnosis, he returned for his annual checkup with his treating oncologist. This time, his lab results were positive. Follow-up tests revealed stage IV melanoma, metastasized to the liver. His cancer had returned with a vengeance.

Casey and his family launched an all-out defensive effort. They consulted a national expert in melanoma treatment and started on an aggressive chemotherapy regimen. By the second round of chemo, Casey was sick with nausea, fatigue, and other side effects. His family was so focused on saving his life that they never stopped to weigh the benefits of care versus cure.

As Casey neared the end of treatment, his tumor markers showed no improvement. Then he developed a bowel obstruction, which required surgery to correct. He felt weak and discouraged. After talking with his oncologist, he decided to stop chemotherapy.

Casey consulted other doctors who had been experimenting with new melanoma protocols. Because his cancer was so widespread, he wasn't eligible for any clinical trials. Much to his family's dismay, he decided to stop treatment altogether. He contacted his local hospice for home care. His goal was to be as comfortable as possible in his last days.

Hospice nurses met with Casey's family to outline their plans for his care. They explained that if Casey rallied and wished to resume treatment, he could do so. He would be welcomed back anytime.

As Casey's condition worsened, his family became more and more frightened. They couldn't cope with his labored talking and his strange breathing noises. They

to the patient but to the patient's loved ones. In fact, hospice actively encourages family members to participate in discussions of a patient's care and to be caregivers themselves.

The Cost of Hospice Care

Often hospice care is less expensive than alternatives such as hospitalization and skilled nursing facilities. Medicare covers hospice services for people who meet its eligibility criteria. So does Medicaid, in 43 states.

If you have private health insurance, reimbursement will depend on your specific health benefits, as well as the level of care you choose. For example, most group plans will pay for in-home hospice visits, as well as for medical equipment rentals such as hospital beds. If you require around-the-clock or even part-time nursing care, you probably will need to cover all or part of the cost. Ninety percent of hospice patients prefer home care, so they can be with their loved ones in familiar surroundings.

Some hospice programs base their fees on

couldn't watch him die, at least not as they had imagined his death.

I knew Casey from previous consultations with him, first around a career transition and then in the anxious period following his original cancer diagnosis. He called to ask if I would make house calls, to help him manage his death and to help his family get through it as well. I agreed.

For the first week, I worked with Casey's family to help them not be afraid of him. The hospice nurses reinforced this message. We taught them how to support this family patriarch who now needed their strong arms and spirits around him.

Eventually, Casey decided that it was time for him to go. He met with his family in my presence, explaining that he had fought as much as he could, that he appreciated their care and concern, and that he loved them. Now he wanted to say good-bye, while he could do so with dignity.

When they argued with him, Casey turned to me and said, "Please help them to let go. It's time. I don't want to be here anymore." He could barely talk. "Please tell them to stop holding back on pain medication from hospice. In the beginning, I asked for less powerful medication so I could be conscious of everything. Now I need more. The pain is getting worse, and I don't want to be so conscious anymore."

I asked Casey's family if they could hear him. They said no, almost in unison. I brought them closer to the bed and asked Casey to repeat his wishes. He barely got out the words, but his family got the message. Two days later, Casey was gone. He had made what was for him the best possible exit.

a patient's ability to pay. Be sure to inquire about this option if it seems appropriate for you.

How to Find Hospice Care

You may choose to enter hospice on your own, or you may receive a referral from a doctor, nurse, social worker, or clergy member. Keep in mind that you always have the option of leaving hospice care, if you wish. In fact, some patients improve to the point that they're able to resume treatment.

To learn more about hospice care, we suggest the following resources.

- Hospice Foundation of America: www.hospicefoundation.org. HFA offers a selection of books, videos, and other materials on hospice care.

- National Hospice and Palliative Care Organization: www.nhpco.org. The site features a search tool to locate hospice services in your area.

DIVISION OF LABOR

TASK	WHO WILL DO IT		
	YOU	PERSONAL ADVOCATE	CPA
1. Assemble your palliative care team.			
2. Find out whether your health insurance provides benefits for hospice care.			
3. Identify hospice services in your area.			

STEP 10

ADDRESS END-OF-LIFE MATTERS

Sometimes, despite the best efforts of the patient and the medical team, cancer is beyond cure. But beyond *cure* doesn't mean beyond *control*. With thought and planning, patients can live out their remaining days in whatever way is desired. That in itself is a victory.

Almost 2 years after his initial diagnosis, Saar was ready to stop fighting his cancer. We had celebrated many victories; for a while, we thought we had won the grand prize—complete remission. Now his cancer was on a rapid march, and Saar's quality of life was slipping below the level that he considered acceptable. He was ready to let go.

I wasn't. I talked Saar into a meeting with one of the consulting experts on his medical team, who—along with our friend Gabe Hortibagyi, MD—advised us of experimental research on a new allogenic transplant procedure. (The term *allogenic* means that the blood cells come from a donor.) Saar's sister and his two children underwent the requisite tests to be donors; of the three, the best candidate was his daughter Laura, who matched him on five of six required markers.

So we had a donor who didn't quite fit the ideal profile and a patient who was slightly past the age limit for the transplant procedure. Despite these issues, the doctors and staff at the M.D. Anderson Cancer Center—where the procedure was in clinical trial—agreed to see us. Before they moved forward, they had a few questions for Saar. Did he know that the mortality rate for procedures at such an early stage of research was 70 percent? Did he know that he would need to stay in Houston for about 3 months to prepare for the transplant? Did he know that he would be in isolation and under constant surveillance for 3 weeks, while they carefully monitored him for signs of graft-versus-host disease?

We had done our research, so Saar was well aware of the risks and drawbacks. He thanked everyone, then said that he would go home and think about the procedure for a couple of days.

Whatever his decision, Saar said, he counted the trip to Houston as another small victory. It allowed him to feel that he had pursued all possible options—even those that I had pushed for and he would have passed on. He was satisfied that he had done all that he could to outwit his cancer.

Eventually, Saar chose not to go ahead with the transplant. The odds against his survival were too great. Even if he did beat the odds, the procedure would buy him just a few extra months. He was willing to trade that time for the energy to be with his family, enjoy them, and say good-bye to them. He wanted to leave this earth with dignity and maybe a few laughs.

Listening to Saar's explanation and seeing his wonderful smile as he contemplated the next life brought a smile to my face as well. I told him that I was fine with his decision.

TIE UP ANY LEGAL OR FINANCIAL LOOSE ENDS

If you haven't taken care of all the paperwork that we discussed in Step 8, now is the time to do so. Your medical designate should receive copies of your advance directives; your legal designate, copies of any important financial documents. Then stow the originals in a safe place—and be sure to tell those who need to know where they are.

The false-bottomed strongbox went out with 19th-century melodrama. For these documents to be of any use, your designates and loved ones must be able to find them. You may assume that your spouse or children already know where you file important papers; perhaps you even showed them at some point in the past. The distress of your illness, or plain forgetfulness, may cause them to overlook even obvious places. Just in case, you may want to make an inventory of key documents and their respective locations. (PCMS Tool #10.1 is perfect for this purpose.)

While you have the physical and mental energy, you may want to think about making your funeral arrangements. Leaving this task for your loved ones could be daunting for them, especially while they're in mourning. Funeral preplanning relieves their burden, while shielding them from information that they really don't need to know. Often preplanning packages cost less, since they're purchased in advance.

If you do have any special requests for your funeral, it's a good idea to discuss them with your spouse or partner, in case any questions arise later on. Also be sure to make a list of people who should be notified of your arrangements.

PCMS Tool #10.1: Keep an Inventory

The following chart includes a list of important documents, with space for you to write down where you've stored them. Make photocopies of the chart—one for your cancer notebook, plus extras for your medical and legal designates, as well as any family members or friends who may need this information. For convenience, you might want to use the following coding system to indicate location.

1. In your home security box

2. In your desk or filing cabinet

3. Someplace else at home (specify location)

4. With your attorney (include name and contact information)

5. With someone else (include name and contact information)

PCMS Tool #10.1	
WHERE THINGS ARE	
DOCUMENTS	LOCATION
Medical—e.g., advance directives, "do not resuscitate" order	
Legal—e.g., will, trusts, estate-planning documents	
Bank account information	
Bill information	
Insurance information	
Funeral arrangements—including a list of whom to notify	
Letters, videos, gifts—for loved ones	

CHOOSE YOUR LIVING ARRANGEMENTS

Some people want to spend the rest of their lives at home; others do not. It's best to communicate your wishes early on and to put those wishes in writing. Cost is a consideration. As suggested in Step 9, you should find out what your health insurance will and won't cover. Among your options:

Hospital: You may feel more comfortable in a setting where medical staff is available and on call around the clock.

Nursing home: If you require supervised care, your insurance policy may dictate that you leave the hospital and enter a nursing home. The primary difference between the two facilities is that in a hospital, you have easier access to physicians as well as available emergency and critical care. If you're not keen on staying in a nursing home, make clear to your personal advocate and loved ones that you'd prefer to transfer to hospice or to stay home, with a private or visiting nurse to provide your care. Where you end up may depend largely on your insurance benefits and your personal resources.

Hospice: Hospice care is available in various settings, including on-site hospice units at hospitals and freestanding hospice facilities. Another option is home hospice services, if you feel strongly about spending your time in the privacy and comfort of your own home. Hospice care is unique in that it addresses the physical, emotional, and spiritual needs of the patient, as well as his or her loved ones. In general, it costs less than a hospital or nursing-home stay. (To learn more about hospice, see Step 9, page 179.)

LIVE WITH DIGNITY

Once you've worked out the logistics of your care, how you spend the rest of your life becomes an issue of values. Some people want to extend their lives as long as they can, using any and all measures to do so. Others focus on quality of life. They'd rather let cancer run its course and do nothing to fight it. Your path is your choice. But once you make that choice, be sure to discuss it with your loved ones, so they honor your request.

Though you may not feel you have the energy for it, make a point of seeing or talking with those closest to you—your children, parents, siblings, and any close friends. This also is the time to write or record any messages to your loved ones. Many of our patients have left letters, videos, and even gifts for the special people in their lives. If you have children, you might wish to leave cards and/or gifts for special occasions such as birthdays, bar mitzvahs, and graduations.

When Saar and I had traveled to Louisville, Kentucky, to visit friends, we had stopped by a shop selling art by local artists. I had admired a pair of green cloth frogs spooning together. For our anniversary, Saar sent for the frogs and gave them to me. We set them on our mantel, where we could look at them in quiet moments during the day. I still do.

PCMS Tool #10.2: Write Your Own Eulogy or Epitaph

This exercise can be deeply rewarding on a personal level. It requires you to think about what your life has meant to you and what you hope it has meant to others. Though you may not feel comfortable sharing such personal information with your family and friends, they're sure to appreciate your message. Ask yourself the following questions.

- What two or three goals did you set for yourself as a young adult?

- What did these goals mean to you?

- What are you most proud of and why?

- What are you least proud of and why?

- What was your happiest time and why?

- Who did you laugh with and why?

- What was your saddest or most painful time and why?

- Who helped you through this time and how?

- Who do you want to talk about and why?

- Do you have a favorite quote or story or film that you want to mention?

SAAR'S GOOD-BYE

At 5:30 p.m. on September 12, 1999, Saar was gone. We buried him at Hillside Memorial Cemetery in Los Angeles the day after his death, in accordance with Jewish tradition. Ever in control, Saar—who had promised to provide the jokes for his funeral—had written his own eulogy, with plenty of punch lines. In his words:

This is a message from the guy in the coffin. Welcome to my family, my friends, and the rest of you. I will keep this short, even though I really have nowhere to go in a hurry.

. . . For years I have been teasing Toni. We buried Mona, Toni's mom, 2 years ago. Mona and I had a tumultuous relationship. My fear is that Toni will get remarried and be buried next to her new husband, and I will be with Mona for eternity. Toni has said that when I meet Mona, she will be young and fun again, so it might not be so bad.

. . . Now for a short announcement. Would the pallbearers please leave their canes and wheelchairs here; we will come back for them. You laugh, but at my age, you have to be concerned. I have been trying to lose weight. Listen, I have chosen two guys who have had angioplasty, one with a total hip replacement, two with bad backs, and one kvetch.

Some of you may feel this is sacrilegious, but I'm afraid that's just me. I also have covered the bases. Not sure that I believe in life after death, I have the Jews here and—thanks to Mitch—the Protestants in Dallas wishing me well.

My simple eulogy message is "Miss me, don't mourn me." I am very fortunate to have lived a good life. I have a wonderful wife; three good kids and their mates; a great sister, Hedria, and her children; family and friends. I have been blessed. I was able to practice the art, not just the science, of medicine. I have been allowed to make a difference. I helped change the way breast disease is treated in LA, the US, and the world. There are women alive today who would not have been otherwise.

I have given tzedakah [to charity].

I have had good, close friends. I have enjoyed life.

Miss me, do not mourn me.

DIVISION OF LABOR

TASK	WHO WILL DO IT		
	YOU	PERSONAL ADVOCATE	CPA
1. Finish any remaining legal and/or financial paperwork.			
2. Make an inventory of important documents using PCMS Tool #10.1.			
3. Weigh your options for living arrangements, and find out which are reimbursable under your health insurance.			
4. Prepare letters, videos, or gifts for your loved ones.			
5. Write your own epitaph or eulogy using PCMS Tool #10.2.			
6. However long you have, live to the end with dignity.			

EPILOGUE

In the course of writing this book, I was diagnosed with cancer. There's nothing like living your subject to make it come alive. I'm pleased to report that today I am considered cured. *I am a cancer survivor.*

No one knows exactly what makes for a cure. It probably is a combination of genetics, biology, and physiology; good doctoring and good (integrative) medicine; a healthy attitude and a wonderful support system; a proactive approach; and a miracle or two. In my case, I practiced what I preached by following the Personal Cancer Management System (PCMS) from day one. I may be biased, but I'm convinced that doing so was a factor in my survival.

As it does for everyone, cancer arrived out of the blue. I'd been having nosebleeds for a couple of months. That wasn't so unusual, since I've had allergies all my life. But when they didn't stop, I'd thought I better investigate.

My first stop was with an ear, nose, and throat (ENT) specialist, who thought the bleeds were "nothing"—perhaps a benign nodule or polyp and some irritated nasal tissue. After a few more weeks, I sought a second opinion from another ENT, Joe Sugarman, MD. He agreed with the first doctor's diagnosis, but he also agreed with my suggestion that a biopsy might be in order. The results showed septal carcinoma. Surgery was required.

Despite the shock, I quickly moved forward by adopting the PCMS. I created my cancer notebook, filled in the medical history chart, and cast a wide net by seeking several medical opinions. I am, by nature, a high-information person; learning everything I could about my diagnosis would help me to feel in control.

Two surgeons later, I was mulling two different opinions. Both surgeons agreed that surgery would be in order, but one said that he'd need to lift up my face in order to see the offending polyp well enough to remove it. He wanted me to schedule the procedure right away. The other felt that he'd be able to reach the polyp by inserting an endoscope in my nose for visibility. He'd give me 2 or 3 weeks to rearrange my schedule. A third surgeon agreed with the second.

Just to be sure, I decided to check with Ken Nieberg, MD, the pathologist who'd made the initial diagnosis. Coincidentally, he was the one who'd found Saar's cancer. When I contacted him, he mentioned that he had been questioning my diagnosis, so he sent my laboratory slides to another pathologist, a specialist, for a second opinion. This time the diagnosis was non-Hodgkins lymphoma (NHL), stage I-EA—E for extranodal, or a visible node, and A for asymptomatic. Instead of surgery, I'd need chemotherapy and radiation.

I reviewed the pathologist's findings with Joe Sugarman, the ENT. He felt that a medical oncologist would be in order and recommended several. I added a few names of my own to the list. I also went online to gather research on my kind of cancer. Ken Schueler, the wonderful research associate for the Porrath Foundation, pointed me to the best resources.

I consulted two medical oncologists, who agreed on the treatment regimen that I would

follow. They and other doctors even used the word *cure*. I was very hopeful.

For my treating oncologist, I chose Edward Wolin, MD, of the recently renamed Samuel Oschin Comprehensive Cancer Institute at Cedars-Sinai Medical Center in Los Angeles. My choice was driven by a number of factors, personal and medical. The institute is an excellent facility, and it's very close to my home and office. Ed Wolin has an excellent reputation, and his opinion was in synch with the others I'd received. He would be able to administer treatment on an outpatient basis, combining IV infusions and a portable chemotherapy pack. This would allow me to continue seeing my own patients and to live as normal a life as possible.

Ed welcomed my input on treatment. For example, he was open to the idea of adding antianxiety medication as well as antiemetic medication to my chemotherapy cocktail to help derail side effects before they started. For the most part, mixing these medicines into the chemo is more effective (though more expensive) than taking them orally. I also consulted a pharmacologist about taking an antidepressant for emotional and immune support.

With my medical team in place, I shifted my focus to assembling my support team. My friend Margot Winchester became my personal advocate, and David Wellish, PhD, became my cancer patient advocate. I was grateful that he'd be available to help me brainstorm ideas, find resources, and make decisions.

Once treatment began, I put together a CAM (complementary and alternative medicine) team consisting of a personal trainer, a chiropractor, and a massage therapist to relieve muscle aches and an acupuncturist to minimize nausea and rebalance my body after the chemotherapeutic toxins did their work. I practiced energy healing and yoga for spiritual support and stress reduction. Mindfulness meditation—sometimes with an instructor—honed my ability to problem-solve.

Halfway through my chemotherapy (three cycles out of six), I scheduled an appointment with Dale Rice, MD, of the USC/Norris Cancer Center in Los Angeles. Dale was one of the surgeons who'd recommended surgery for the nasal polyp. Since he had seen the polyp full-blown, he could tell whether or not it was responding to treatment. With a simple test, Dr. Rice pronounced the polyp gone. He even mentioned that wonderful word: *cure*.

Both Dale and Peter Rosen, MD, a medical research oncologist at UCLA Medical Center and my local expert on non-Hodgkins lymphoma, concluded that I had received enough chemotherapy and should switch to radiation. But Ed Wolin, my treating oncologist, was reluctant to stop chemo, since I was in the middle of a six-cycle protocol. Another doctor recommended five cycles of chemo with no radiation.

I was becoming very weak from treatment, and my hemoglobin count was looking rather puny. I had been getting booster shots to elevate those numbers and tests to keep tab on the results. But I'd been neglecting to check the results; when I did, I realized that the numbers had gotten away from me. My body was yelling, "Stop!" What to do?

As the PCMS advises, once all of the research and opinions are in, the patient must make the decisions. I considered all the treatment options that my medical team had presented to me. Another factor was a recent scan that showed a possible problem with my pancreas. Though everyone believed it to be a technical glitch with the scan—an overcall or a false positive, which isn't uncommon—I decided to go for a fourth round of chemotherapy, along with an endoscopic ultrasound with biopsy to take a direct look at my pancreas. It turned out to be perfectly healthy.

So after four cycles of chemotherapy, I called it quits. Ed Wolin was reluctant to break with his original protocol, but ultimately he agreed. Then I was faced with another decision, this time about the radiation protocol. Two radiation oncologists, two opinions—different techniques, different dosages, different durations. Once again I did my research and consulted my cancer patient advocate, David Wellish. I opted for the shorter course. My radiation oncologist was Ron Thompson, MD, who by coincidence had treated Saar at Cedars-Sinai, where he had been chief of radiation oncology for most of his career.

Five weeks later, at my posttreatment checkup, I was pronounced cured. I wish I could say that put a period on cancer for me, and I haven't thought about it since. But right now, forgetting seems impossible. I still see each of my doctors on a regular basis. I still update my records in my cancer notebook. I worry about every blemish and muscle ache in a way I never did before. It will be awhile before cancer becomes a back-of-mind thing for me. I doubt it ever will leave my mind for good.

Just as the PCMS recommends, I have been working to rebuild my body, mind, and spirit. I continue to follow my CAM regimen—though with few adjustments, since it's more of a wellness program now. I relax more. I laugh more. I see my family more. My hair is thicker and curlier, thanks to chemotherapy. I am thinner and working to stay that way. I've become closer to the wonderful friends and family who stood by me, especially my children. And every day I work to build my belief and faith in that marvelous word *cure*.

Life does feel wonderful again.

RESOURCES

FINDING INFORMATION ONLINE

The Internet can be a valuable resource for staying on top of the very latest developments in cancer diagnosis and treatment. Finding authoritative, trustworthy information is critical. We've created this guide to help you navigate the online universe, so you can find what you need—and weed out what you don't. Many of the Web sites here appear elsewhere in the book as well. We've collected them in one place for easy reference.

Searching Smart

Before you begin any search, you need to find a reliable search tool, one that specializes in health and medical information. The most precise are evaluated subject catalogs, which drive you to Web sites that have been prescreened by health professionals. Among the most highly regarded are the following:

- Hardin MD
  www.lib.uiowa.edu/hardin/md

Provides easy access to cancer information.

- HealthWeb
  www.healthweb.org

An index of evaluated noncommercial, health-related online resources of interest to health professionals and researchers, as well as to consumers.

- MedWeb
  www.medweb.emory.edu/MedWeb

A catalog of biomedical and health-related Web sites maintained by the staff of the Robert W. Woodruff Health Sciences Center Library at Emory University.

Other search engines are great for providing a general overview of what's available online. They don't prescreen search results, so you need to do some investigating on your own. The more popular engines include:

- Alltheweb
  www.alltheweb.com

- AltaVista
  www.altavista.com

- Google
  www.google.com

- Wisenut
  www.wisenut.com

- Yahoo
  www.yahoo.com

Some search engines, like Google and Yahoo, arrange their information into categories. You can click through the categories until you find what you need.

Another search option is the metasearch engine, which browses multiple search engines at the same time. Because metasearches concentrate on the big picture, they can miss information that a "regular" search engine would find. For this reason, we don't recom-

mend relying on metasearch engines exclusively. Two to check out:

- Dogpile
  www.dogpile.com

- MetaCrawler
  www.metacrawler.com

Your best bet is to choose one or two search engines and learn all of their unique features. This will maximize the effectiveness of your search. But if you don't find what you need with one search engine, try another. They don't overlap as much as you might expect.

Remember to vary the word order in your search. For example, "non-Hodgkin's lymphoma" might generate different results than "lymphoma, non-Hodgkin's." Also use synonyms; if you're looking for information on "pulmonary lymphoma," type in related words such as "lung" or "respiratory."

Because of the way search engines select and organize their search results, you are most likely to find what you need in the first 50 "hits." Looking through more than that is probably a waste of time.

Screening Sites

The Internet puts a wealth of information at your fingertips. It does have certain limitations, however. Separating reliable from unreliable sources is a major concern, especially for health topics like cancer. Anyone can post anything online. An official-looking Web site doesn't guarantee the accuracy or legitimacy of the content.

Look for Web sites that bear the imprimatur HONCODE, indicating that they subscribe to the principals of the Health on the Net Foundation. And when you visit a site, be sure to ask the questions that follow.

Who is responsible for maintaining the site? Every Web address, or URL, has a three-letter extension known as a domain name. The most common domain names are:

- com (for-profit company)
- edu (educational institution)
- gov (government agency)
- org (nonprofit organization)

In general, Web sites that use "edu" or "gov" are good resources, though some educational institutions allow students to post personal Web pages. Sites with the "com" or "org" designation can be reputable as well, but they may be worth a background check if you don't recognize the sponsoring organization. A site that's run by a for-profit company most likely is selling something, which may skew any research or information they offer.

Is the information current? Breakthroughs in cancer diagnosis and treatment happen constantly. You want to make sure that you have the very latest information. Check when a Web site received its last update. Usually you can find a date at the bottom of the Web page, with a note such as "posted date," "last updated," or "page last modified."

Does advertising totally support the Web site? Be wary of sites that post large banner ads or that use "brought to you by . . . " or some similar tagline. Any site that depends on advertising for all of its financial support may present biased information.

Our Top Picks

From our work with cancer patients and through our own cancer experience, we've amassed a collection of Web sites that we feel comfortable recommending. All have authoritative sponsoring organizations, and all stay abreast of advances and trends in cancer diagnosis and treatment. This list is not all-inclusive; feel free to supplement it with your own favorite sites, as you wish.

General Cancer Information

- American Cancer Society (ACS) www.cancer.org

Offers information and tools for finding clinical trials, exploring treatment options, making treatment decisions, and more. Can search by zip code for ACS resources in your area.

- Association of Cancer Online Resources www.acor.org

Provides access to free, unmoderated discussion groups for cancer patients, family and friends, physicians, and researchers.

- Cancer*Care* www.cancercare.org

Offers free support services—including education, counseling, physician referrals, and financial assistance—to cancer patients and their loved ones.

- National Cancer Institute's Center for Cancer Research ccr.nci.nih.gov/news/

An excellent resource for keeping up with ongoing research developments and for checking newspaper databases.

• R.A. Bloch Cancer Foundation
www.blochcancer.org

An advocacy organization for cancer patients and their caregivers; its hotline is staffed by trained cancer survivors.

Clinical Trials

• Abramson Cancer Center of the University of Pennsylvania
oncolink.upenn.edu

Matches cancer patients to clinical trials; also allows you to post questions to cancer experts.

• Coalition of Cancer Cooperative Groups
www.cancertrialshelp.org

Provides a tool for locating clinical trials specific to your type of cancer.

• National Institutes of Health
www.clinicaltrials.gov

Directs you to federally and privately funded clinical studies accepting human volunteers.

• Rational Therapeutics
www.rationaltherapeutics.com

An independent research laboratory that specializes in cancer treatment protocols tailored to the patient.

• Sidney Kimmel Comprehensive Cancer Center at Johns Hopkins
www.hopkinskimmelcancercenter.org

Allows you to search ongoing clinical trials by cancer type. The center also sponsors education and community outreach initiatives.

• Stanford Hospital and Clinics
http://www.stanfordhospital.com/clinicsmedServices/index.html

Click on "Oncology" for information about ongoing clinical trials, as well as specific cancers.

• Thomson CenterWatch
www.centerwatch.com

Offers a listing of ongoing clinical trials by medical specialty, including oncology.

Online Consultations and Second Opinions

• Cleveland Clinic
www.eclevelandclinic.org

Offers remote second opinions from Cleveland Clinic experts, who will review your medical records and diagnostic tests.

• Partners Online Specialty Consultations
www.econsults.partners.org

A health care consultation service that provides second opinions to physicians on behalf of their patients.

• University of Texas M.D. Anderson Cancer Center
www.mdanderson.org

Offers outside consultation pathology services, which provide second opinion evaluation of tissue samples submitted by physicians and pathologists on behalf of cancer patients.

Pain Management

- American Pain Foundation
  www.painfoundation.org

A nonprofit organization whose goal is to increase awareness of and bring an end to the undertreatment of pain. Provides links to support groups, along with other pain management resources.

- American Pain Society
  www.ampainsoc.org

Advocates on behalf of pain management research and education; offers online and print information on cancer pain.

- Elsevier
  www.elsevier.com

The home of Elsevier, which publishes several medical journals on pain management and offers online access to journal articles.

Medications

- Amgen
  www.Amgen.com

Amgen manufactures Epogen and Neulasta, both of which help alleviate chemotherapy-related side effects. Visit the Web site for information on the company's patient assistance program, which provides medications for underinsured and uninsured patients.

- Ortho Biotech
  www.procrit.com

Procrit is a prescription medication that alleviates chemotherapy-related anemia and resulting fatigue. The manufacturer, Biotech, offers prescription assistance to qualified patients.

- *Physicians' Desk Reference*
  www.pdr.net

Profiles hundreds of prescription and over-the-counter medications. Requires registration to use.

Psychological and Emotional Support

- American Psychosocial Oncology Society
  www.apos-society.org

Offers an online directory of counselors and other support providers who specialize in psychosocial cancer care.

- International Psycho-Oncology Society
  www.ipos-society.org

Provides links to online patient forums and support groups, as well as ordering information for a number of print publications.

- The Wellness Community
  www.thewellnesscommunity.org

This Washington, DC–based nonprofit organization sponsors support groups and educational programs for cancer patients and their families.

Complementary and Alternative Therapies

- National Center for Complementary and Alternative Medicine (NCCAM) nccam.nih.gov

Under the auspices of the National Institutes of Health, NCCAM supports scientific research to validate the therapeutic benefits of various complementary and alternative disciplines.

- Richard and Hinda Rosenthal Center for Complementary and Alternative Medicine www.rosenthal.hs.columbia.edu

The mission of the Rosenthal Center, affiliated with the Columbia University College of Physicians and Surgeons, is to foster the responsible study and practice of complementary and alternative therapies. The site provides descriptions of ongoing clinical trials.

Legal, Financial, and Workplace Issues

- Cancer Legal Resource Center (CLRC) http://wlcdr.everybody.org/special-programs/cancer.html

A joint program of Loyola Law School and the Western Law Center for Disability Rights, CLRC offers consultations on the full spectrum of legal issues that can affect cancer patients.

- Caring Connections www.caringinfo.org

Offers information about advance care planning and financial planning, among other topics.

- Health Insurance Information, Counseling, and Assistance Program http://www.hiicap.state.ny.us/index.htm

Sponsored by the New York State Office for the Aging, this site provides links to other state-sponsored health insurance programs.

- Patient Advocate Foundation www.patientadvocate.org

A national nonprofit organization that acts as a liaison to resolve issues between cancer patients and their insurers or employers.

- Social Security Administration www.ssa.gov

Explains federal guidelines for collecting disability benefits. You can apply for benefits online.

- US Living Will Registry www.uslivingwillregistry.com

Provides state-specific forms for advance directives and stores them for distribution on 24 hours' notice.

Palliative Care and Hospice Services

- Hospice Foundation of America www.hospicefoundation.org

Offers information and resources for end-of-life care.

- Hospice Institute for Education, Training, and Research
  www.hospice.com

Provides an overview of hospice and physician-assisted living.

- National Hospice Foundation
  www.nationalhospicefoundation.org

Features a tool to search for hospice facilities by state or zip code.

- National Hospice and Palliative Care Organization
  www.nhpco.org

Helps locate resources for a variety of end-of-life matters, including palliative care, hospice, and home health care.

For Cancer Survivors

- California Cancer Registry
  www.ccral.org

Features links to cancer survivor Web pages and online support groups.

- Cancer Survivors Online
  www.cancersurvivors.org

Sponsors online chats and message boards, plus links to other resources.

- National Cancer Survivors Day Foundation
  www.ncsdf.org

Provides information on the issues that affect cancer survivors.

- National Coalition for Cancer Survivorship
  www.canceradvocacy.org

A survivor-led advocacy organization that promotes quality cancer care for all Americans.

INDEX

Boldface page references indicate illustrations.
Underscored references indicate boxed text.